DENGUE - IMMUNOPATHOLOGY AND CONTROL STRATEGIES

Edited by **Márcia Aparecida Sperança**

Dengue - Immunopathology and Control Strategies
http://dx.doi.org/10.5772/65522
Edited by Márcia Aparecida Sperança

Contributors
Andrew W Taylor-Robinson, Narayan Gyawali, Leopoldo Flores-Romo, Edith Marcial-Juárez, Juan Carlos Yam-Puc, Leticia Cedillo-Barrón, Juana Calderón-Amador, Raúl Antonio Maqueda-Alfaro, Nonantzin Beristain-Covarrubias, Alejandro Escobar-Gutiérrez, Julio García-Cordero, Karina Ruiz-Tovar, Mariana Orozco-Uribe, Ming-Kung Yeh, Yuan-Chuan Chen, Hwei-Fang Cheng, Yi-Chen Yang, Shamaraz Firdous, Shahzad Anwar, Youichi Suzuki, Hirotaka Takahashi, Pablo Manrique-Saide, Azael Che-Mendoza, Josue Herrera-Bojorquez, Josue Villegas-Chim, Guillermo Guillermo-May, Anuar Medina-Barreiro, Felipe Dzul-Manzanilla, Abdiel Martin-Park, Gabriela Gonzalez-Olvera, Juan Ignacio Arredondo-Jiménez, Adriana Flores-Suarez, Norma Pavia-Ruz, Catrin Huws Jones, Gonzalo Vazquez-Prokopec, Audrey Lenhart, Hugo Delfin-Gonzalez, Ambreen Zubair, Asim Ahmed, Jorge Abelardo Falcón-Lezama, Roberto Tapia-Conyer, Miguel Betancourt-Cravioto

Published by InTech
Janeza Trdine 9, 51000 Rijeka, Croatia

Publishing Process Manager Marijana Francetic
Technical Editor SPi Global
Cover InTech Design team

First published July, 2017
Printed in Croatia
Legal deposit, Croatia: National and University Library in Zagreb

Additional hard copies can be obtained from orders@intechopen.com

Dengue - Immunopathology and Control Strategies, Edited by Márcia Aparecida Sperança
p. cm.
Print ISBN 978-953-51-3435-0
Online ISBN 978-953-51-3436-7

For EU product safety concerns:
IN TECH d.o.o., Prolaz Marije Krucifikse Kozulić 3, 51000 Rijeka, Croatia,
info@intechopen.com or visit our website at intechopen.com.

Meet the editor

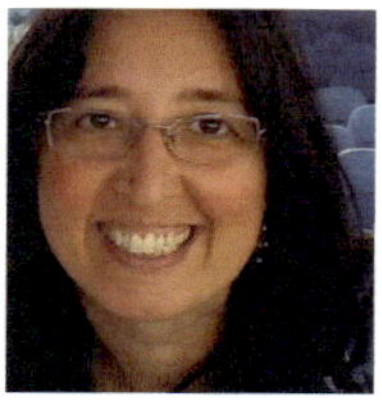

Márcia Aparecida Sperança serves as an associate professor at the Center for Natural and Human Sciences of the Universidade Federal do ABC (UFABC, São Bernardo do Campo, São Paulo, Brazil). After getting a PhD degree in Biology of Parasite-Host Interaction at Parasitology Department of Biomedical Science Institute of University of São Paulo (Brazil), she worked as an assistant professor and researcher at Marilia Medical School (Marilia, São Paulo, Brazil). Her scientific experience is in diagnosis, molecular biology, and molecular epidemiology of different infectious agents including arboviruses, the bacteria *Helicobacter pylori*, malaria parasites, and trypanosomatids. Presently, Dr. Sperança is the head of the Laboratory of Pathogenic Agents at UFABC, an institution with multi- and interdisciplinary academic proposals, which are characteristics of her investigation field.

Contents

Preface

Dengue is the most prevalent arthropod-borne virus in the tropical and subtropical areas of the world being transmitted by mosquitoes from genus *Aedes*, principally the highly wide-reaching *A. aegypti* and *A. albopictus*. Dengue virus (DENV) is present in four serotypes (DENV1–4) with genetic intraserotypic variation. Multiple dengue serotypes co-circulation lead to increasing risk for recombination and this occurs in subtropical and tropical regions. Natural history of DENV indicates that all serotypes circulating in the world originated from a single ancestor and dispersed from sylvatic forests of Africa and Asia, where the recently new serotype DENV5 was isolated. DENV5 was restricted to an outbreak occurred in 2007 in a sylvatic area of Malaysia and thus is not included as a global serotype.

All DENV serotypes are associated to different clinical manifestations ranging from asymptomatic, nonspecific flu-like symptoms and classical expression (high fever, headache, pain behind the eyes, muscle and joint pains, rash) to severe hemorrhagic dengue fever and shock syndrome due to exacerbation in immunologic response resulting in high decrease in platelets and plasma leakage. Risk for severe dengue fever increases in heterotypic secondary infection, a phenomenon described as ADE (antibody-dependent enhancement), which is one of the principal drawbacks in dengue vaccine development. Therefore, a correct diagnosis with monitoring of serotypes and its genetic variation is of great importance to the management of different clinical manifestations associated to DENV and also to a vaccine implementation.

In the end of 2015, a tetravalent recombinant dengue vaccine developed by Sanofi Pasteur (CYD-TDV, Dengvaxia®), which presents as the backbone of the yellow fever-attenuated live vaccine, was licensed in Mexico. The efficiency of this vaccine is low (and varies according to serotypes and in different regions) being recommended by the World Health Organization only to regions with high burden of disease. Thus, until an efficient vaccine can be developed, the main strategy to manage DENV corresponds to vector control with participation of community.

In this scenario, the edited book *Dengue - Immunopathology and Control Strategies* contains eight chapters divided in three sections that underline the important aspects of DENV, including virus replication cycle and pathology, diagnostic methods, and control. The first section brings knowledge on the basic aspects of dengue virus replication which can be associated to its immunopathology. The first chapter focuses on cellular factors involved in DENV infection and viral replication modulation, including a description of molecular and cellular tools to be used in identification and description of new factors associated to DENV replication. In order to comprehend the mechanism of ADE, in Chapter 2, the natural in vivo route of DENV was assessed from the entrance of the virus via the skin until its arrival and distribution inside regional draining lymph nodes and its potential association with antigen-presenting cells. Participation of the liver in the pathology of DENV was approached in Chapter 3.

The second section includes two chapters on dengue diagnosis and emphasizes that in spite of the many scientific efforts, this subject continues to be a drawback in the disease control. Chapter 4 corresponds to a review on strong and weak aspects of available DENV diagnostic methods and a prospect for its improvements. Development of optical DENV diagnostic tests employing spectroscopy is shown in Chapter 5.

Vector-based control strategies are discussed in the third section of the book, in Chapter 6. The authors reveal the utility of insecticide-treated houses in the reduction of *A. aegypti* population in a Latin American region. Chapters 7 and 8 correspond to, respectively, a description on regulation of dengue vaccines and the experience of Mexico in the implementation of the unique registered dengue vaccine.

Hopefully, this book will bring valuable information about dengue disease basic aspects, immunopathology, and diagnostic and control strategies to a broad public including undergraduate and postgraduate students, researchers from different knowledge areas, and health professionals. I am grateful to all authors for their precious contributions and to InTech Corporation for the opportunity to participate as an editor of a book on this important global life-threatening disease.

Márcia Aparecida Sperança, PhD
Center for Natural and Human Sciences
Federal University of ABC
Campus São Bernardo do Campo
São Paulo, Brazil

Section 1

Virus Replication Cycle and Pathology

Chapter 1

Cellular Control of Dengue Virus Replication: Role of Interferon-Inducible Genes

Hirotaka Takahashi and Youichi Suzuki

Additional information is available at the end of the chapter

http://dx.doi.org/10.5772/67984

Abstract

Dengue, one of the most common mosquito-borne viral infectious diseases in the world, is caused by the dengue virus (DENV). This enveloped RNA virus has immunologically distinct serotypes that increase the risk of life-threatening diseases, such as dengue haemorrhagic fever. However, no effective antiviral therapy against DENV infection has yet been established. As seen in other RNA viruses, various cellular factors have been reported to participate in efficient DENV replication. On the other hand, increasing recent evidence demonstrates that host cells harbour inhibitory factors that limit the DENV replication. In particular, it is well known that the response of interferons (IFNs), the first line of a host defence system against invading pathogens, evokes the expression of a number of genes that negatively regulate various steps of virus replication. This set of inhibitory genes, called interferon-stimulated genes (ISGs), is considered to be a central force in IFN-mediated antiviral responses. In this chapter, we focus our attention on the cellular factors involved in DENV infection, particularly to those that modulate DENV replication through their association with viral RNA. In addition, we also summarize general experimental approaches for identifying the host factors of RNA viruses, including DENV.

Keywords: dengue virus, cellular factors, RNA untranslated regions, interferon-stimulated genes, identification systems

1. Introduction

Dengue virus (DENV) is an enveloped and positive-strand RNA virus that belongs to the genus *Flavivirus* of the Flaviviridae family [1]. An important characteristic of the Flavivirus is that this genus consists of a large number of arthropod-borne viruses, many of which are transmitted by mosquitoes and ticks. In addition, flavivirus infection often causes life-threatening diseases in humans, such as haemorrhagic fever, encephalitis, and meningitis [2]. Recently, the Zika virus (ZIKV), a member of the flavivirus family that has spread explosively throughout the Americas, is reported to be associated with neurological complications [3, 4]. Flaviviruses, therefore, have significant clinical as well as economic impacts on modern society.

DENV is a mosquito-borne virus widely distributed in the tropical and subtropical areas of the world. This flavivirus infection is transmitted to humans via the bite of infected mosquitos. The primary vector of DENV infection is *Aedes aegypti,* while *Aedes albopictus,* which originated in Asia but has extended its range to other regions of the world, is also capable of spreading a dengue outbreak. DENV has four antigenically distinct serotypes (from DENV-1 to DENV-4). Primary infection with one of the serotypes is often asymptomatic or causes self-limiting dengue fever (DF). However, secondary infection of different serotypes increases the risk of more serious forms of DENV infection, such as dengue haemorrhagic fever (DHF) and dengue shock syndrome (DSS), due to the presence of non- or sub-neutralizing antibodies generated during the primary infection. Therefore, dengue is a significant threat to humans, yet there is currently no specific antiviral available for DENV infection [1, 5]. However, it should be noted that a live attenuated vaccine against DENV developed by Sanofi Pasteur (Dengvaxia) has been licensed for use in a limited number of countries, including Mexico and the Philippines, although the efficacy of the DENV vaccine in endemic countries is still under investigation [6].

2. Brief overview of DENV replication

DENV infection begins with its entry into a permissive cell via receptor-mediated endocytosis (**Figure 1**). So far, various types of human cells, such as macrophages, lymphocytes, hepatocytes, and endothelial cells, are reportedly susceptible to DENV infection. Among them, monocyte lineage cells (i.e., dendritic cells [DCs] and macrophages) are thought to be the primary targets of DENV in humans. As the entry receptors of DENV, several cellular proteins, including C-type lectin receptors (e.g., DC-SIGN/CD209, mannose receptor/CD206) and phosphatidylserine receptors (e.g., TIM, TAM), have been demonstrated [7].

Upon entry into the cell, a membrane fusion between DENV envelope (E) glycoprotein and endosomal vesicle occurs, leading to the release of viral RNA into the cytoplasm. The DENV genome is a single-stranded positive-sense RNA and is approximately 10-kb long. The viral RNA contains a single long open reading frame (ORF) flanked by highly structured 5′ and 3′ untranslated regions (UTRs), with a type 1 cap (m7GpppAmp) at the 5′ terminus and no poly(A) tract at the 3′ terminus [8]. The single ORF is translated to a large polyprotein, which is subsequently cleaved co- and post-translationally into three structural (capsid [C], pre-membrane [prM], and E) and seven non-structural (NS) proteins (NS1, NS2A, NS2B, NS3, NS4A, NS4B, and NS5) by viral (NS3) and host proteases (**Figure 1A**). Of the NS proteins, NS5, the largest viral protein, functions as an RNA-dependent RNA polymerase (RdRp), which synthesizes a complementary minus-strand RNA template and, in turn, produces many copies of

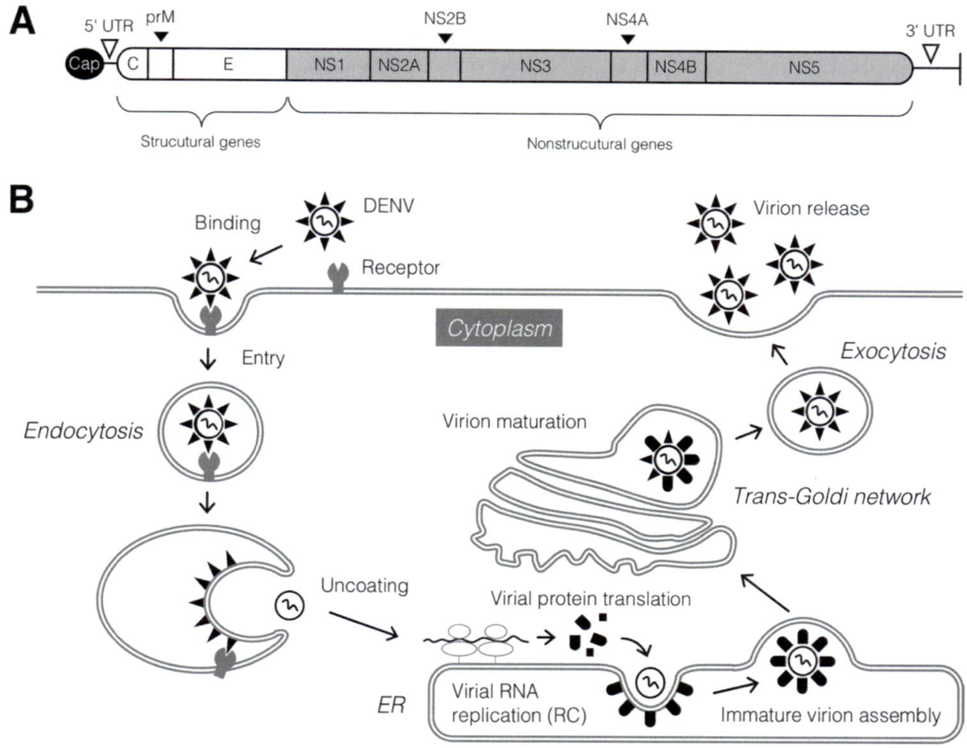

Figure 1. The genome structure and replication cycle of DENV.

positive-strand viral genomic RNA. Viral RNA replication takes place in the so-called replication complexes (RCs) composed of viral RNA and proteins as well as hypothetical cellular proteins, which are formed on the endoplasmic reticulum (ER) membrane. This membrane structure, rearranged by DENV infection, is also the place of viral RNA translation, protein processing, and progeny virion assembly [9]. The immature particles then bud into the ER lumen and are transported through the secretion pathway of the trans-Golgi network, in which progeny virions undergo a maturation process via a conformational change of prM and E proteins on the virion surface. Finally, mature, infectious virions egress from infected cells by exocytosis (**Figure 1B**) [5, 8].

3. Cellular factors involved in DENV replication: interaction with viral RNA untranslated regions

As seen in other RNA and DNA viruses, flaviviruses, including DENV, have been shown to utilize biological processes of the host to replicate efficiently in infected cells through the interaction between viral and cellular proteins. Although the biological relevance of many of the host interactors in *in vivo* replication and the pathogenicity of DENV remain unclear, those virus-host interactions could serve as attractive targets of antiviral drugs [2]. In addition to the entry receptors, intracellular factors implicated in the replication cycle of DENV have been comprehensively reviewed elsewhere [2, 8, 10, 11]. Meanwhile, it is becoming apparent that various cellular cofactors are recruited into the 5′ and 3′ UTRs of DENV RNA, which results in enhanced virus replication [12].

The DENV 5′ and 3′ UTRs are approximately 100 and 350–700 nucleotides long, respectively (**Figure 1A**). The primary sequences located within or adjacent to the UTRs have been shown to be essential for virus replication [8]. For instance, complementary sequences, termed CS (cyclization sequence) elements, found in the ORF of capsid and the 3′ UTR and UAR (upstream of the AUG region) elements, found in the 5′ and 3′ UTRs, are reported to physically anneal to mediate DENV genome cyclization. This cyclization is likely to recruit the DENV RdRp at the 5′ end of the viral genome and then likely to facilitate viral RNA amplification [13]. Additionally, DENV UTRs form stable secondary and tertiary structures, and these structural integrities are thought to be important for the regulation of viral RNA synthesis and translation process. Therefore, albeit the sequences are diverse, UTR secondary structures are highly conserved among flaviviruses [8]. Furthermore, these regions have been demonstrated to contain several cellular proteins [12].

An early study that employed an *in vitro*-formed nucleoprotein complex of synthesized DENV 3′ UTR and mosquito cell extracts identified some RNA-binding proteins—the La autoantigen, translation elongation factor-1α (EF-1α), and polypyrimidine tract-binding protein (PTB)—as the DENV UTR-associated cellular factors in cells [14]. Subsequent studies have also revealed that human La protein binds not only with the DENV 3′ UTR but also with the 5′ UTR [15, 16]. Interestingly, interactions of La protein with viral proteins NS3 and NS5 were shown, suggesting that the La protein is somehow involved in the function of RC in infected cells [15]. The La autoantigen is reported to associate with RNA polymerase III transcription; interestingly, this RNA-binding protein has also been shown to stimulate the translation of viral and cellular mRNAs by binding with their UTRs [17]. As with mosquito EF-1α, its human homologue (i.e., EF1A) has been reported to specifically recognize the conserved 3′-terminal stem-loop (SL) in the 3′ UTR of West Nile virus (WNV) RNA [18]. Given the colocalization of EF-1α with the DENV RC in the infected cell [19], it can be suggested that this cellular protein also plays an important role in the function of flaviviral RNA. However, the precise step of flaviviral replication in which EF-1α is involved remains to be elucidated [19].

PTB is a ubiquitous RNA-binding protein known to be involved in splicing, polyadenylation, stability, and translation of cellular mRNA [20]. With regard to its role in virus infection, PTB has been shown to bind to the UTRs of picornaviruses [21, 22] and the hepatitis C virus (HCV) [23]; it functions as an internal ribosome entry site, (IRES)-trans-acting factor, to activate viral translation [24, 25]. On the other hand, several studies have raised questions about the involvement of PTB in the translation process of those RNA viruses [26–28]. Interestingly, both La and PTB were implicated in HCV replication [29]. In the case of DENV infection, PTB is reportedly required for efficient replication. Furthermore, PTB interacted with a DENV protein, NS4, as well as viral RNA, suggesting that PTB associates with DENV RCs [30]. Although it remains unclear whether PTB regulates DENV RNA simplification or the translation process (or another step of virus infection), PTB may function as a molecular chaperone to stabilize the structured viral RNA [30, 31]. In addition to the host factors mentioned above, recent studies using tobramycin RNA aptamer affinity chromatography identified DDX6 (DEAD-box RNA helicase) and ERI3 (putative 3′–5′ RNA exonuclease) as DENV UTR-binding cellular proteins that promote DENV replication [32, 33].

The genome of flaviviruses, including DENV, encodes enzymes required for viral RNA synthesis (i.e., RdRp and helicase) and viral protein processing (i.e., protease); however, the viral protein translation process must rely fully on the translational machinery of the host [34], except for the methyltransferase activity conferred by NS5, which adds a type 1 7-methylguanosine cap to the 5′ terminus of viral RNA. It is, therefore, not surprising that cellular factors are associated with DENV RNA during viral translation [8, 35]. At the initiation step of eukaryotic mRNA translation, a 5′ cap structure is first recognized by a eukaryotic initiation factor, eIF4E, which, in turn, leads to the recruitment of eIF4G. eIF4G serves as a scaffold protein that binds the DEAD-box RNA helicase eIF4A and also the poly(A)-binding protein (PABP), resulting in the circularization of mRNA [8]. This complex formation induces the association of the 43S ribosomal subunit through the binding of the eIF3 complex. Finally, the 60S ribosomal subunit joins the initiation complex that enables the elongation process of translation [8]. In the case of DENV, its genomic RNA is 5′ capped but lacks 3′-end poly(A) sequences [8]. Nevertheless, PABP is shown to interact with DENV 3′ UTR *in vitro* by recognizing the A-rich regions upstream of 3′ SL in the 3′ UTR [36]. Indeed, a study using chimeras reported that mRNA based on a cellular (globin) gene and DENV RNA revealed that DENV 3′ UTR exhibits functions similar to those of polyadenylated non-viral UTRs in enhancing translation rather than RNA stabilization [37]. Thus, it is plausible that as with cellular mRNA, translated DENV RNA also forms a closed-loop structure via association with host translation factors [38]. In addition, it is demonstrated that DENV RNA may be able to produce proteins by a 5′ cap-independent translation mechanism in certain cellular situations in which the eIF4E is starved and, thereby, canonical host translation is inhibited [39].

4. Experimental procedures for identifying the cellular factors

In the following sections, we summarize several general approaches to search for the cellular factors involved in virus infections.

4.1. Conventional methods using living cells

4.1.1. Gene expression analysis and proteomic analysis

Studies using a microarray system, quantitative RT-PCR analysis, and GeneChip analysis have revealed that the expression levels of many mRNAs in host cells are dramatically altered upon DENV infection [40–42]. It is highly possible that some of these DENV-responsible genes and their products function as crucial positive or negative regulators of DENV replication in cells. Indeed, tumour necrosis factor–related apoptosis-inducing ligand (TRAIL), whose mRNA expression level significantly increased with DENV infection, was found to be a negative regulator of DENV replication [42]. In addition to the analysis of the gene expression profile, the global host protein expression profile upon DENV infection was also investigated by comprehensive proteomic analysis. Conventionally, the total host proteins extracted from infected cells and control cells were separated by two-dimensional PAGE (2-D PAGE), and the proteins whose expression levels were altered by the viral infection were picked up, and their amino acid sequences were determined with mass spectrometry (MS) analysis. Previous studies have identified many host factors that respond to DENV infection [43, 44]. More recently, a proteomic analysis based on stable isotope labelling by amino acids in cell culture (SILAC), which overcame the limitations of sensitivity and resolution of 2-D PAGE, was developed and applied to DENV research [45, 46]. The technologies of high-throughput gene expression analysis and proteomic analysis are thought to be powerful tools for understanding the global cellular expression profile of host cells upon DENV infection, both at the gene and at the protein levels. From the results of these assays alone, however, it is difficult to distinguish whether DENV-responsible host factors that are identified are indeed involved in the regulation of viral replication. To understand the roles and functions of these hit factors requires further functional analysis.

4.1.2. RNAi screening

RNA interference (RNAi) is a well-known approach for identifying novel host factors in virus-infected cells. When the knockdown of a host gene by RNAi alters the efficiency of viral replication, it is highly possible that this gene works as a host factor of the virus. Currently, commercial siRNA pools that cover most human genes are available, and many genome-wide comprehensive screenings for many kinds of viruses have been performed thus far [47–49]. In studies of flaviviruses, hundreds of host factor proteins involved with the early steps of WNV infection have been identified by silencing more than 20,000 human genes from a small interfering RNA (siRNA) pool [50]. An additional bioinformatic study, followed by the siRNA screening, revealed that many of these hits were involved in the ubiquitin-proteasome pathway and the ER-associated degradation (ERAD) pathway, both of which are essential for many steps of viral replication. In addition to host factors in human cells, one study aimed to identify host factors from insect cells, another host of DENV [51]. In that study of DENV-adapted cells from *Drosophila melanogaster* and an siRNA pool targeting more than 20,000 genes of *Drosophila*, the proteins that accelerate or inhibit the replication of DENV in *Drosophila* cells were identified [51]. Then human analogues of hit genes in *Drosophila* cells were subsequently silenced in DENV-infected human cultured cells, and 42 of these were found to be common host factors in human and *Drosophila* cells [51]. It is noteworthy that RNAi screening can identify host factors that can affect viral replication either by direct interaction with viral components or by indirect interaction, such as the regulation of the IFN pathway.

4.1.3. Yeast two-hybrid analysis

For researchers attempting to identify host factors that directly interact with viral proteins, yeast two-hybrid (Y2H) analysis is a common and effective way; numerous host factors of many viruses, including DENV, have been identified using this system [52–58]. Taking advantage of good throughput, several large screenings were performed to build DENV host interactomes using human cDNA libraries. One study reported that a Y2H analysis using either partial or full-length DNA fragments encoding each DENV protein and the human liver cDNA library identified 105 viral-host interactions; further knockdown experiments using siRNAs revealed that six proteins were essential for the efficient viral replication of DENV [59]. Another study also carried out a Y2H assay using NS3 and NS5 proteins from DENV and other flaviviruses as bait, and 108 human proteins were identified as interacting with NS3 or NS5 or both [60]. In addition, Y2H assays were performed to identify DENV proteins interacting with host factors from human and mosquito cDNA libraries. They identified several common host factors conserved in both humans and mosquitos [61]. These studies identified many host proteins that interact with DENV proteins; however, few of the hits overlap in independent studies. Although this might be caused mainly by the fact that the assay in each study was performed in different conditions and with different cDNA libraries, it is also possible that each study includes many false positives and false negatives.

4.2. Wheat germ–based protein array system

4.2.1. Overview of the protein array technology

As described above, the living cell-based methods are powerful tools for identifying viral-host interactions since the assays could be carried out under physiological conditions, at least partially. However, these methods have several disadvantages. First, proteins whose expression levels are quite low or that show cytotoxicity are hard to analyse. Second, immunoprecipitation assays are commonly used to detect the interaction between a protein and a protein; however, the number of interactions that can be detected at one time is limited. Therefore, it is highly possible that many researchers have potentially overlooked important but difficult-to-detect interactions in their first screenings using living cells. To solve these problems, we recently developed a novel biochemical screening method based on a wheat germ cell–free protein synthesis system (wheat cell-free system) and high-throughput binding assay. The wheat cell-free system enables the synthesis of various kinds of eukaryotic proteins in a 96-well format [62]. So far, proteins having several transmembrane domains, relatively large molecular weights, and cytotoxic activity were successfully synthesized by this system [63, 64]. This robust protein synthesis system allows us to establish a "protein array", from which tens to thousands of recombinant proteins sorted by their functions were arrayed into each well of a 96-well plate [65]. The protein arrays currently available in our research group are shown in **Table 1** [65–70]. Based on these protein arrays, we have established a high-throughput binding assay for identifying proteins directly bound to target proteins from the array. To perform hundreds to tens of thousands of binding reactions, a luminescent-based binding assay, called AlphaScreen, was employed [65, 66, 71]. This assay is able to use crude translation products of wheat cell-free synthesis to detect binding reactions by mixing these crude proteins in a 384-well plate, followed by adding two beads and the antibody for detection. Because of its flexibility, AlphaScreen can be used not only as a binding assay but also as a protein cleavage assay for a viral protease. The principle of the assays is shown in **Figure 2**.

Protein array	Origin	Number of proteins	References
Protein kinase	Human and mouse	400	Masaki et al. [66], Miyakawa et al. [67], Kudoh et al. [68]
E3 ligase	Human and mouse	250	Takahashi et al. [65], Tan et al. [69]
Deubiquitinating enzyme	Human	85	Unpublished
Single transmembrane protein	Human and mouse	730	Unpublished
Auto-antigen protein	Human and mouse	2100	Matsuoka et al. [70]

Table 1. Wheat cell–free-based protein arrays currently available in our research group.

4.2.2. Practical applications for viral research

We and other research groups have done several assays using this technology to identify host proteins that interacted with viral proteins. In researching the HCV (a virus related to DENV), several protein kinases were found to bind directly with the HCV non-structural protein NS5A using the protein kinase array; by phosphorylating NS5A through additional functional analysis using a cultured cell system, one protein kinase, Casein kinase I-α, was found to regulate viral replication [66]. The protein kinase array was used to identify other host factors that

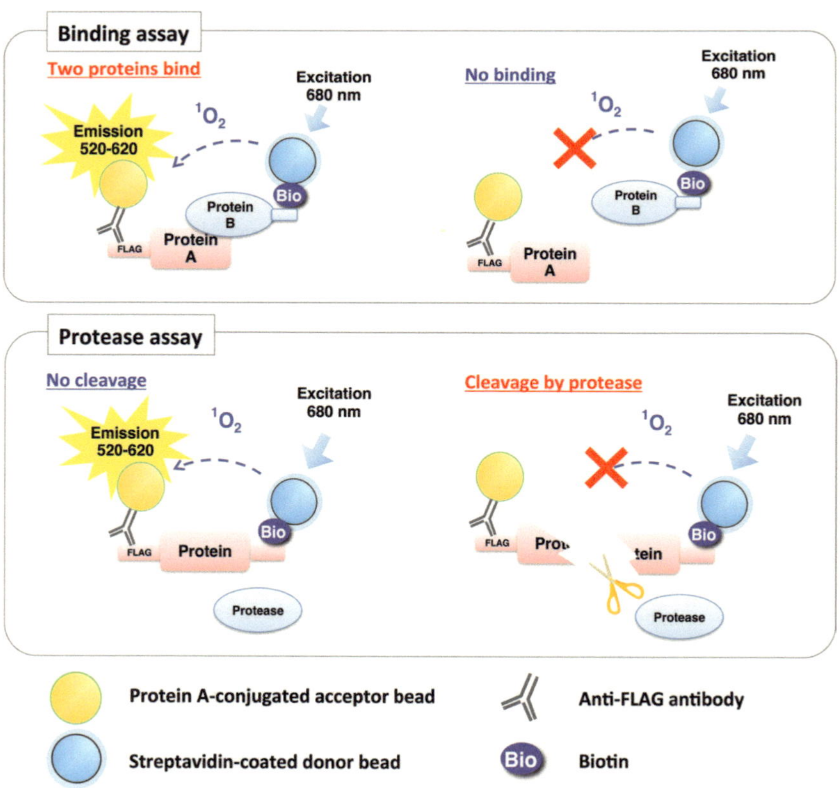

Figure 2. A schematic diagram of binding assay and protease assay based on AlphaScreen technology.

functionally interacted with human immunodeficiency virus (HIV) proteins [67, 68]. In the case of the protease assay, one research article demonstrated that a protease from xenotropic murine leukaemia virus-related virus (XMRV) and 24 cellular proteins that were target candidates of the viral protease were synthesized; *in vitro* cleavage assay revealed several novel substrates of XMRV protease [72], indicating the feasibility of using wheat cell–free-based protein array technology and high-throughput biochemical assay based on AlphaScreen.

4.2.3. Wheat cell–free protein array for DENV research

Thus far, NS3 and NS5 proteins of DENV have been considered difficult to synthesize as full-length active recombinant proteins using a conventional protein expression system, such as for *Escherichia coli*. We previously reported that the wheat cell-free system successfully synthesized full-length NS3 and NS5 proteins in a soluble form; some biochemical analyses revealed that both recombinant proteins possessed enzymatic activities [63], indicating the usefulness of the expression system for the preparation of DENV proteins. In addition to these soluble proteins, NS4B, a protein with at least three transmembrane domains, was synthesized with the wheat cell-free system (**Figure 3A**). Our preliminary study demonstrated that NS4B was

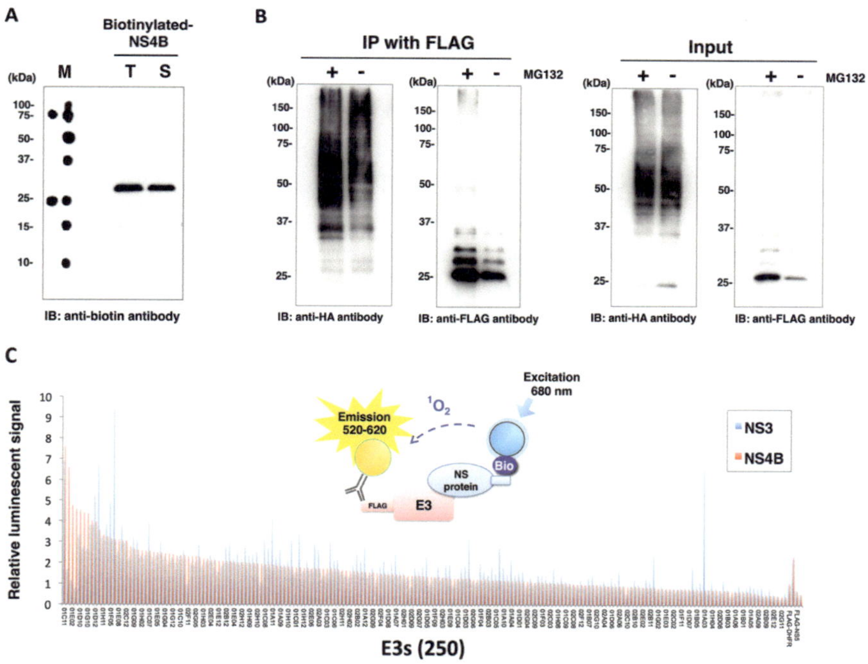

Figure 3. Identification of E3 ligases targeting DENV NS4B by wheat cell-free-based protein array system. (A) Expression of biotinylated NS4B with wheat cell-free system. The total translation products of NS4B (T) and supernatant (S) after centrifugation of the total translation product were subjected to SDS-PAGE, followed by immunoblot analysis using anti-biotin antibody. M is the molecular marker. (B) Ubiquitination of NS4B. HEK293T cells overexpressing FLAG-tagged NS4B and HA-tagged ubiquitin were treated with proteasomal inhibitor MG132, and FLAG-tagged NS4B was precipitated with anti-FLAG antibody. The NS4B and ubiquitin were detected by immunoblot analysis using anti-FLAG antibody and anti-HA antibody, respectively. (C) AlphaScreen assay to identify the E3s targeting DENV NS3 and NS4B proteins using the E3 protein array. Biotinylated NS3 and NS4B were used as bait, and biotinylated DHFR was used as negative control of NS proteins. The relative luminescent signal was calculated as follows: the value from E3 and NS4B/value from E3 and DHFR.

highly ubiquitinated when NS4B was overexpressed in HEK293T cells (**Figure 3B**), suggesting that the amount of NS4B expressed was regulated in host cells in a ubiquitin/proteasome-dependent manner. When a protein is ubiquitinated and, subsequently, degraded by the 26S proteasome, E3 is a determinant of the ubiquitination, as E3 specifically binds to the target protein and transfers activated ubiquitin from the ubiquitin conjugation enzyme, E2 [73]. Therefore, we screened NS4B-binding E3s from the E3 protein array using AlphaScreen, as we recently reported [65]. NS3 was used as control to determine the NS4B-specific E3s. As shown in **Figure 3C**, many E3s were found to bind with recombinant NS4B. Currently, additional functional analysis, such as *in vitro* ubiquitination assay and protein degradation assay in cells, is ongoing.

5. Restriction of DENV infection by cellular inhibitors

As previously mentioned, DENV hijacks the host's biological process for its efficient replication. Meanwhile, it has become apparent that DENV infection can be limited by cellular factors. In this sense, the innate immune response induced by IFN is considered to be the first line of defence against DENV [8]

Generally, RNA viruses that infect target cells are sensed by the pattern recognition receptors (PRRs), which specifically recognize a component of invading viruses. As for DENV infection, the membrane-bound Toll-like receptors (TLR3, TLR7, TLR8) and the cytosolic receptors (retinoic acid-inducible gene I [RIG-I], melanoma differentiation-associated gene 5 [MDA5]) are reported to be the PRRs for viral RNA [74–77]. These recognitions in turn activate adaptor molecules of the PRR, leading to the activation of a downstream phosphorylation cascade and the subsequent production of IFN and pro-inflammatory cytokines (**Figure 4**) [78]. Among the IFNs produced, type I IFNs, including IFNα, IFN-β, and IFN-ω, play an important role in antiviral immunity [79]. The type I IFN then binds to its receptors (IFNAR) on neighbouring cells and signals to induce the phosphorylation of signal transducers and the activators of transcriptions 1 and 2 (STAT1 and 2) in cytoplasm. This phosphorylation of STAT1/2 triggers the formation of IFN-stimulated gene factor 3 (ISGF3) with IFN-regulatory factor 9 (IRF9). Finally, the ISGF3 complex translocates to the nucleus and acts as a transcription activator for the expression of a number of genes by binding to the IFN-stimulated response elements (ISREs) on chromosomes (**Figure 4**) [80].

As seen above, IFN is considered to be an inducer of the antiviral state, and it has been well demonstrated that actual antiviral effector molecules in the IFN response are a subset of the genes upregulated by IFN, which are called IFN-stimulated genes (ISGs). Thus far, hundreds of genes have been classified as ISGs, and many of them are reported to have inhibitory effects on divergent families of viruses, including flaviviruses [80–83]. Importantly, several ISGs have also been shown to restrict DENV infection, and their suppressive effects are likely to be exerted at the multiple steps of virus replication, including virus entry (IFITMs [84, 85], ADAP2 [86]), viral RNA/protein synthesis (ISG20 [87], viperin [88, 89]), and infectious virion production (tetherin [90], ISG15 [91, 92]). In addition, a comprehensive study using an over-expression of a cDNA library derived from known ISGs demonstrates the involvement of

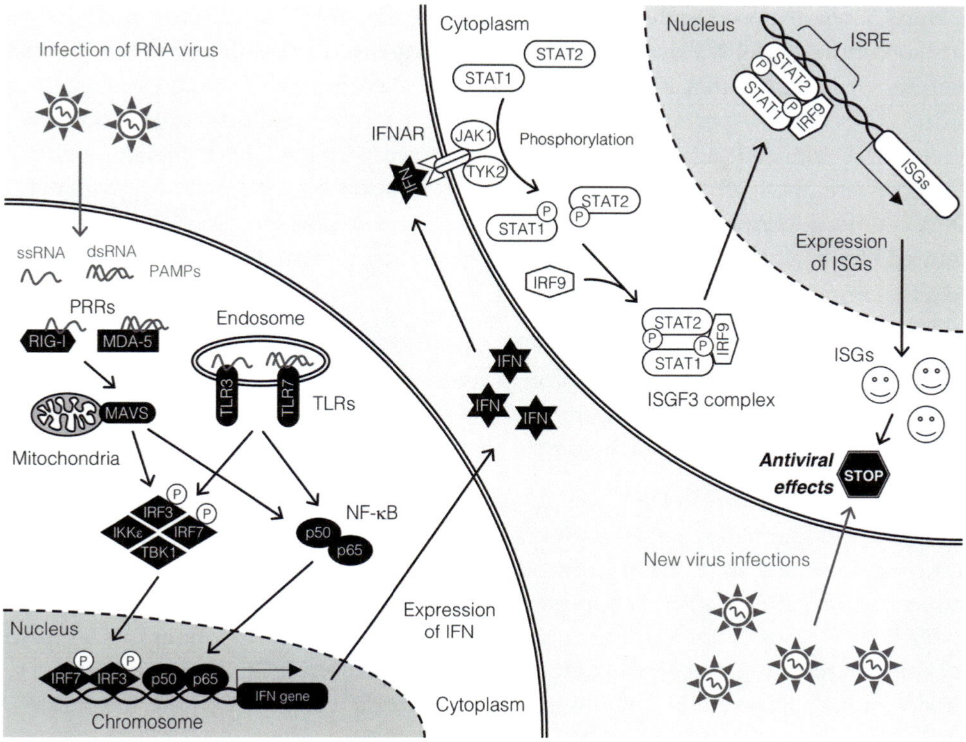

Figure 4. Intracellular recognition of RNA viruses and IFN responses (left). PRRs-sensing virus-specific nucleic acid structures (ssRNA and dsRNA) activate signalling cascades via phosphorylation of transcription factors (IRF3 and IRF7), which leads to the expression of IFN genes together with NF-κB (right). Binding of IFNs produced from virus-infected cells to type I IFN receptor (IFNAR) activates JAK1 and TYK2, which, in turn, phosphorylate STAT1 and STAT2. Phosphorylation of STAT1/2 induces the formation of ISGF3 complex with IRF9, and finally, ISGF3 translocated in nucleus binds to ISREs to induce ISG expressions. ssRNA, single-stranded RNA; dsRNA, double-stranded RNA; MAVS, mitochondrial antiviral-signalling protein; JAK1, Janus kinase 1; and TYK2, tyrosine kinase 2.

many more ISGs in the restriction of DENV [93]. However, the precise mechanisms of these ISG-mediated anti-DENV activities remain unclear, and we will have to wait for future studies for detailed analysis.

6. Identification of RyDEN/C19orf66 as novel anti-DENV ISG

It has been well demonstrated that a gain-of-function (i.e., overexpression) screen of cDNA is a powerful approach to identifying antiviral ISGs [82, 83, 93, 94]. In a recent study, we employed the gain-of-function strategy using a pool of cDNA library derived from type 1 IFN-treated cells to search for ISGs suppressing DENV replication in human cells [95]. In this approach, a human cervical carcinoma cell line, HeLa, was treated with type I IFN (a mixture of human IFN-α and -ω) for 24 hours at a concentration that had been reported to inhibit DENV infection *in vitro* [96], and mRNA from the IFN-treated HeLa cells was converted into a library of cDNA and transferred to a HIV-based lentiviral vector. Then, a human hepatoma cell line, Huh7.5, was exposed to the HIV vector carrying the IFN cDNA library. Huh7.5 cells are highly susceptible to DENV and, therefore, exhibit massive cell death upon DENV infection. Therefore, we expected that if anti-DENV genes derived from IFN-treated HeLa cells were introduced into DENV-permissive Huh7.5 cells, those cells should be non-permissive and survive DENV-induced cell death. As anticipated, even with the DENV challenge, surviving cell clones were obtained; subsequent sequencing analysis revealed that approximately half of DENV-resistant clones harboured an ORF of a gene on chromosome 19, *C19orf66*, in the integrated HIV vector genome [95]. Since *C19orf66* was a previously uncharacterized gene, we named this *r*epressor of *y*ield of *DEN*V (RyDEN).

The ORF of RyDEN (*C19orf66*) encodes a 291 amino acid protein, and the secondary structure prediction suggested that the RyDEN protein contained a nuclear localization signal (NLS) in the middle region and a nuclear export signal (NES) in the C-terminal region. Additionally, a characteristic glutamic acid (E)-rich domain was found in the C-terminus.

The anti-DENV activity of RyDEN was confirmed by creating stable cell lines that expressed epitope tag-fused human hepatoma cell lines, and all DENV serotypes (i.e., DENV-1–4) were found to be inhibited by RyDEN expressions. In line with the fact that this gene was first identified by the gain-of-function approach using an IFN-derived cDNA library, expressions of RyDEN in various human cell lines were upregulated by IFN treatment to a greater or lesser extent, indicating that RyDEN is a bona fide anti-DENV ISG. More importantly, when the endogenous expression of RyDEN mRNA was knocked down by RNAi, the suppressive activity of type I IFNs against DENV became less effective, suggesting that RyDEN was a major contributor of the IFN-mediated anti-DENV response [95].

One question to ponder: what is the molecular mechanism by which RyDEN suppresses DENV replication? Affinity purification-mass spectrometry analysis with affinity tag-fused RyDEN found that RyDEN interacted with two other cellular proteins, poly(A)-binding protein cytoplasmic 1 (PABPC1) and La motif-related protein 1 (LARP1). PABPC1 is a member of the PABP family; as described above, this protein bridges the 5′ and 3′ ends of mRNA by binding both the eIF4G and the poly(A) tail, which stimulates the initiation of translation [97]. LARP1 is also an RNA-binding protein and one of the LARPS, which shares the signature motif with the La autoantigen, called the La motif (LM). Therefore, Larp and La proteins are categorized as being in the same family [98]. Intriguingly, LARP1 is shown to interact with PABP to stimulate the mRNA translation process [99, 100]. Considering the positive effect of PABP on translation [97], the association of PABPC1 and LARP1 with RyDEN suggests that RyDEN might interfere with the translation of DENV RNA by inhibiting PABPC1 and LARP1 functions. Indeed, this speculation was supported by the following findings: (i) an RNAi-mediated knockdown of PABPC1 and LARP1 significantly reduced the level of DENV replication, (ii) PABPC1 interacted with DENV RNA in infected cells, (iii) the expression of RyDEN suppressed the expression of the reporter protein from a DENV-based sub-genomic RNA replicon that lacked structural (C, prM, E) genes, and (iv) the recruitment of RyDEN to the DENV RNA 3′ UTR was enhanced by the presence of PABPC1 *in vitro* [95]. Therefore, one could envisage that the anti-DENV activity of RyDEN, an antiviral ISG, is exerted during the translation of viral RNA by associating PABPC1/LARP1 with the 3′ UTR and somehow interfering with the function of the translation factors (**Figure 5**). Or another possibility is that

http://dx.doi.org/10.5772/67984

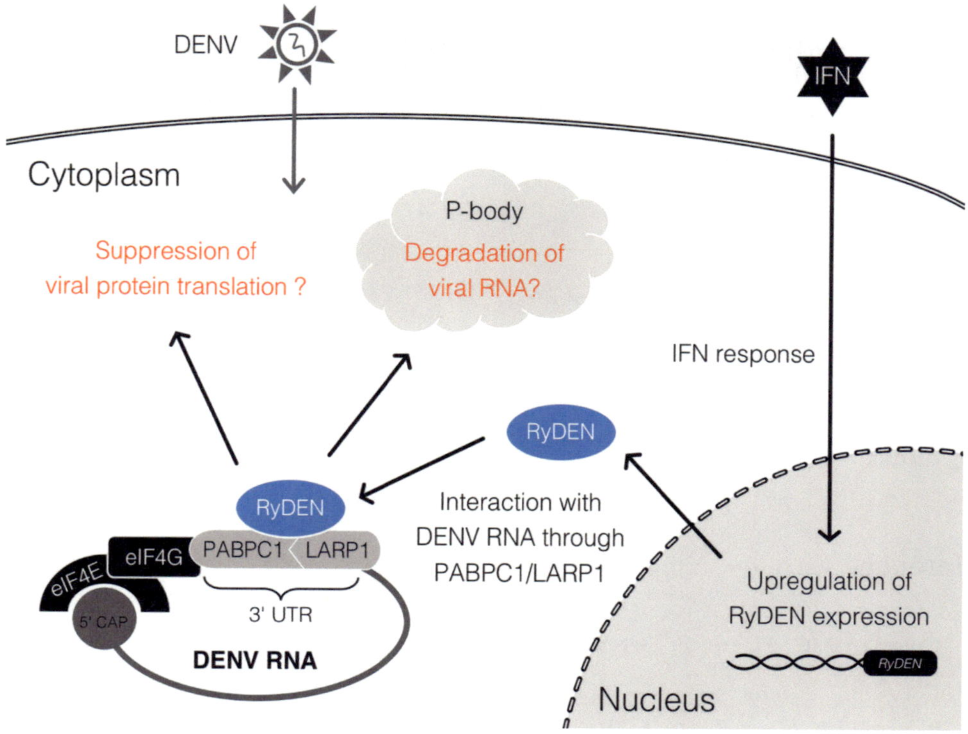

Figure 5. Possible mechanisms by which RyDEN restricts the function of DENV RNA. RyDEN, whose expression is upregulated by IFN, associates with DENV RNA through interaction with PABPC1 and LARP1 that are required for DENV replication. This association may result in (i) translational suppression or (ii) degradation of viral RNA in the cytoplasm.

RyDEN may facilitate the degradation of viral RNA, since PABPC1 and LARP1 have been reported to be involved in eukaryotic mRNA decay as processing body (P-body) and stress granule (SG) components (**Figure 5**) [99, 101]. In accordance with this notion, a recent study revealed that RyDEN (also referred to as FLJ11286 or IRAV) was colocalized with cytoplasmic P-bodies in IFN-treated cells [102]. Furthermore, it was noteworthy that RyDEN expression limited a diverse range of RNA and DNA viruses [83, 95, 102], indicating that RyDEN is a broad-spectrum antiviral ISG.

7. Concluding remarks

This chapter highlighted the molecular interactions between DENV and host factors, particularly focused on the cellular regulation of DENV replication. As is well known, IFN response is one of the host controls of DENV infection and pathogenesis [96, 103, 104]. Although the effector molecules in the IFN response that actually interfere with virus replication remain fully clarified, profound efforts have been made to identify the IFN-inducible cellular factors restricting RNA virus replication, including DENV [80]. It should be noted that antagonistic effects of DENV infection on IFN signalling and production, which are mediated by several means using viral factors, are observed [105–107]. However, the characterization of anti-DENV ISGs is to illuminate the "heel of Achilles" of DENV, which will provide the underpinnings for the development of antivirals against dengue.

Author details

Hirotaka Takahashi[1] and Youichi Suzuki[2]*

*Address all correspondence to: californiacircle@gmail.com

1 Proteo-Science Center, Ehime University, Matsuyama, Japan

2 Department of Microbiology and Infection Control, Osaka Medical College, Takatsuki, Japan

References

[1] Guzman MG, Harris E. Dengue. Lancet. 2015;**385**:453-465. doi:10.1016/S0140-6736(14)60572-9

[2] Pastorino B, Nougairede A, Wurtz N, Gould E, de Lamballerie X. Role of host cell factors in flavivirus infection: implications for pathogenesis and development of antiviral drugs. Antiviral Research. 2010;**87**:281-294. doi:10.1016/j.antiviral.2010.04.014

[3] Basarab M, Bowman C, Aarons EJ, Cropley I. Zika virus. BMJ. 2016;**352**:i1049. doi:10.1136/bmj.i1049

[4] Becker R. Missing link: animal models to study whether Zika causes birth defects. Nature Medicine. 2016;**22**:225-227. doi:10.1038/nm0316-225

[5] Diamond MS, Pierson TC. Molecular insight into dengue virus pathogenesis and its implications for disease control. Cell. 2015;**162**:488-492. doi:10.1016/j.cell.2015.07.005

[6] Villar L, Dayan GH, Arredondo-Garcia JL, Rivera DM, Cunha R, Deseda C, Reynales H, Costa MS, Morales-Ramirez JO, Carrasquilla G, Rey LC, Dietze R, Luz K, Rivas E, Miranda Montoya MC, Cortes Supelano M, Zambrano B, Langevin E, Boaz M, Tornieporth N, Saville M, Noriega F, Group CYDS. Efficacy of a tetravalent dengue vaccine in children in Latin America. New England Journal of Medicine. 2015;**372**:113-123. doi:10.1056/NEJMoa1411037

[7] Perera-Lecoin M, Meertens L, Carnec X, Amara A. Flavivirus entry receptors: an update. Viruses. 2013;**6**:69-88. doi:10.3390/v6010069

[8] Clyde K, Kyle JL, Harris E. Recent advances in deciphering viral and host determinants of dengue virus replication and pathogenesis. Journal of Virology. 2006;**80**:11418-11431. doi:10.1128/JVI.01257-06

[9] den Boon JA, Diaz A, Ahlquist P. Cytoplasmic viral replication complexes. Cell Host Microbe. 2010;**8**:77-85. doi:10.1016/j.chom.2010.06.010

[10] Fischl W, Bartenschlager R. Exploitation of cellular pathways by Dengue virus. Current Opinion in Microbiology. 2011;**14**:470-475. doi:10.1016/j.mib.2011.07.012

[11] Krishnan MN, Garcia-Blanco MA. Targeting host factors to treat West Nile and dengue viral infections. Viruses. 2014;**6**:683-708. doi:10.3390/v6020683

[12] Bidet K, Garcia-Blanco MA. Flaviviral RNAs: weapons and targets in the war between virus and host. Biochemical Journal. 2014;**462**:215-230. doi:10.1042/BJ20140456

[13] Villordo SM, Gamarnik AV. Genome cyclization as strategy for flavivirus RNA replication. Virus Research. 2009;**139**:230-239. doi:10.1016/j.virusres.2008.07.016

[14] De Nova-Ocampo M, Villegas-Sepulveda N, del Angel RM. Translation elongation factor-1alpha, La, and PTB interact with the 3′ untranslated region of dengue 4 virus RNA. Virology. 2002;**295**:337-347. doi:10.1006/viro.2002.1407

[15] Garcia-Montalvo BM, Medina F, del Angel RM. La protein binds to NS5 and NS3 and to the 5′ and 3′ ends of Dengue 4 virus RNA. Virus Research. 2004;**102**:141-150. doi:10.1016/j.virusres.2004.01.024

[16] Yocupicio-Monroy RM, Medina F, Reyes-del Valle J, del Angel RM. Cellular proteins from human monocytes bind to dengue 4 virus minus-strand 3′ untranslated region RNA. Journal of Virology. 2003;**77**:3067-3076.

[17] Bousquet-Antonelli C, Deragon JM. A comprehensive analysis of the La-motif protein superfamily. RNA. 2009;**15**:750-764. doi:10.1261/rna.1478709

[18] Blackwell JL, Brinton MA. Translation elongation factor-1 alpha interacts with the 3′ stem-loop region of West Nile virus genomic RNA. Journal of Virology. 1997;**71**:6433-6444.

[19] Davis WG, Blackwell JL, Shi PY, Brinton MA. Interaction between the cellular protein eEF1A and the 3′-terminal stem-loop of West Nile virus genomic RNA facilitates viral minus-strand RNA synthesis. Journal of Virology. 2007;**81**:10172-10187. doi:10.1128/JVI.00531-07

[20] Romanelli MG, Diani E, Lievens PM. New insights into functional roles of the polypyrimidine tract-binding protein. International Journal of Molecular Sciences. 2013;**14**:22906-22932. doi:10.3390/ijms141122906

[21] Hellen CU, Witherell GW, Schmid M, Shin SH, Pestova TV, Gil A, Wimmer E. A cytoplasmic 57-kDa protein that is required for translation of picornavirus RNA by internal ribosomal entry is identical to the nuclear pyrimidine tract-binding protein. Proceedings of the National Academy of Sciences of the United States of America. 1993;**90**:7642-7646.

[22] Jang SK, Wimmer E. Cap-independent translation of encephalomyocarditis virus RNA: structural elements of the internal ribosomal entry site and involvement of a cellular 57-kD RNA-binding protein. Genes and Development. 1990;**4**:1560-1572.

[23] Ito T, Lai MM. An internal polypyrimidine-tract-binding protein-binding site in the hepatitis C virus RNA attenuates translation, which is relieved by the 3′-untranslated sequence. Virology. 1999;**254**:288-296. doi:10.1006/viro.1998.9541

[24] Jang SK. Internal initiation: IRES elements of picornaviruses and hepatitis c virus. Virus Research. 2006;**119**:2-15. doi:10.1016/j.virusres.2005.11.003

[25] Martinez-Salas E, Pacheco A, Serrano P, Fernandez N. New insights into internal ribosome entry site elements relevant for viral gene expression. Journal of General Virology. 2008;**89**:611-626. doi:10.1099/vir.0.83426-0

[26] Aizaki H, Choi KS, Liu M, Li YJ, Lai MM. Polypyrimidine-tract-binding protein is a component of the HCV RNA replication complex and necessary for RNA synthesis. Journal of Biomedical Science. 2006;**13**:469-480. doi:10.1007/s11373-006-9088-4

[27] Choi KS, Huang P, Lai MM. Polypyrimidine-tract-binding protein affects transcription but not translation of mouse hepatitis virus RNA. Virology. 2002;**303**:58-68.

[28] Tischendorf JJ, Beger C, Korf M, Manns MP, Kruger M. Polypyrimidine tract-binding protein (PTB) inhibits Hepatitis C virus internal ribosome entry site (HCV IRES)-mediated translation, but does not affect HCV replication. Archives of Virology. 2004;**149**:1955-1970.

[29] Domitrovich AM, Diebel KW, Ali N, Sarker S, Siddiqui A. Role of La autoantigen and polypyrimidine tract-binding protein in HCV replication. Virology. 2005;**335**:72-86. doi:10.1016/j.virol.2005.02.009

[30] Anwar A, Leong KM, Ng ML, Chu JJ, Garcia-Blanco MA. The polypyrimidine tract-binding protein is required for efficient dengue virus propagation and associates with the viral replication machinery. Journal of Biological Chemistry. 2009;**284**:17021-17029. doi:10.1074/jbc.M109.006239

[31] Karakasiliotis I, Chaudhry Y, Roberts LO, Goodfellow IG. Feline calicivirus replication: requirement for polypyrimidine tract-binding protein is temperature-dependent. Journal of General Virology. 2006;**87**:3339-3347. doi:10.1099/vir.0.82153-0

[32] Ward AM, Bidet K, Yinglin A, Ler SG, Hogue K, Blackstock W, Gunaratne J, Garcia-Blanco MA. Quantitative mass spectrometry of DENV-2 RNA-interacting proteins reveals that the DEAD-box RNA helicase DDX6 binds the DB1 and DB2 3′ UTR structures. RNA Biology. 2011;**8**:1173-1186. doi:10.4161/rna.8.6.17836

[33] Ward AM, Calvert ME, Read LR, Kang S, Levitt BE, Dimopoulos G, Bradrick SS, Gunaratne J, Garcia-Blanco MA. The Golgi associated ERI3 is a flavivirus host factor. Scientific Reports. 2016;**6**:34379. doi:10.1038/srep34379

[34] Jackson RJ, Hellen CU, Pestova TV. The mechanism of eukaryotic translation initiation and principles of its regulation. Nature Reviews: Molecular Cell Biology. 2010;**11**:113-127. doi:10.1038/nrm2838

[35] Li MM, MacDonald MR, Rice CM. To translate, or not to translate: viral and host mRNA regulation by interferon-stimulated genes. Trends in Cell Biology. 2015;**25**:320-329. doi:10.1016/j.tcb.2015.02.001

[36] Polacek C, Friebe P, Harris E. Poly(A)-binding protein binds to the non-polyadenylated 3′ untranslated region of dengue virus and modulates translation efficiency. Journal of General Virology. 2009;**90**:687-692. doi:10.1099/vir.0.007021-0

[37] Chiu WW, Kinney RM, Dreher TW. Control of translation by the 5′- and 3′-terminal regions of the dengue virus genome. Journal of Virology. 2005;**79**:8303-8315. doi:10.1128/JVI.79.13.8303-8315.2005

[38] Edgil D, Harris E. End-to-end communication in the modulation of translation by mammalian RNA viruses. Virus Research. 2006;**119**:43-51. doi:10.1016/j.virusres.2005.10.012

[39] Edgil D, Polacek C, Harris E. Dengue virus utilizes a novel strategy for translation initiation when cap-dependent translation is inhibited. Journal of Virology. 2006;**80**:2976-2986. doi:10.1128/JVI.80.6.2976-2986.2006

[40] Liew KJ, Chow VT. Differential display RT-PCR analysis of ECV304 endothelial-like cells infected with dengue virus type 2 reveals messenger RNA expression profiles of multiple human genes involved in known and novel roles. Journal of Medical Virology. 2004;**72**:597-609. doi:10.1002/jmv.20034

[41] Warke RV, Xhaja K, Martin KJ, Fournier MF, Shaw SK, Brizuela N, de Bosch N, Lapointe D, Ennis FA, Rothman AL, Bosch I. Dengue virus induces novel changes in gene expression of human umbilical vein endothelial cells. Journal of Virology. 2003;**77**:11822-11832.

[42] Warke RV, Martin KJ, Giaya K, Shaw SK, Rothman AL, Bosch I. TRAIL is a novel antiviral protein against dengue virus. Journal of Virology. 2008;**82**:555-564. doi:10.1128/JVI.01694-06

[43] Higa LM, Caruso MB, Canellas F, Soares MR, Oliveira-Carvalho AL, Chapeaurouge DA, Almeida PM, Perales J, Zingali RB, Da Poian AT. Secretome of HepG2 cells infected with dengue virus: implications for pathogenesis. Biochimica et Biophysica Acta. 2008;**1784**:1607-1616. doi:10.1016/j.bbapap.2008.06.015

[44] Kanlaya R, Pattanakitsakul SN, Sinchaikul S, Chen ST, Thongboonkerd V. The ubiquitin-proteasome pathway is important for dengue virus infection in primary human endothelial cells. Journal of Proteome Research. 2010;**9**:4960-4971. doi:10.1021/pr100219y

[45] Chiu HC, Hannemann H, Heesom KJ, Matthews DA, Davidson AD. High-throughput quantitative proteomic analysis of dengue virus type 2 infected A549 cells. PLoS One. 2014;**9**:e93305. doi:10.1371/journal.pone.0093305

[46] Viktorovskaya OV, Greco TM, Cristea IM, Thompson SR. Identification of RNA binding proteins associated with dengue virus RNA in infected cells reveals temporally distinct host factor requirements. PLoS Neglected Tropical Diseases. 2016;**10**:e0004921. doi:10.1371/journal.pntd.0004921

[47] Zhou H, Xu M, Huang Q, Gates AT, Zhang XD, Castle JC, Stec E, Ferrer M, Strulovici B, Hazuda DJ, Espeseth AS. Genome-scale RNAi screen for host factors required for HIV replication. Cell Host Microbe. 2008;**4**:495-504. doi:10.1016/j.chom.2008.10.004

[48] Brass AL, Dykxhoorn DM, Benita Y, Yan N, Engelman A, Xavier RJ, Lieberman J, Elledge SJ. Identification of host proteins required for HIV infection through a functional genomic screen. Science. 2008;**319**:921-926. doi:10.1126/science.1152725

[49] Tai AW, Benita Y, Peng LF, Kim SS, Sakamoto N, Xavier RJ, Chung RT. A functional genomic screen identifies cellular cofactors of hepatitis C virus replication. Cell Host Microbe. 2009;**5**:298-307. doi:10.1016/j.chom.2009.02.001

[50] Krishnan MN, Ng A, Sukumaran B, Gilfoy FD, Uchil PD, Sultana H, Brass AL, Adametz R, Tsui M, Qian F, Montgomery RR, Lev S, Mason PW, Koski RA, Elledge SJ, Xavier RJ, Agaisse H, Fikrig E. RNA interference screen for human genes associated with West Nile virus infection. Nature. 2008;**455**:242-245. doi:10.1038/nature07207

[51] Sessions OM, Barrows NJ, Souza-Neto JA, Robinson TJ, Hershey CL, Rodgers MA, Ramirez JL, Dimopoulos G, Yang PL, Pearson JL, Garcia-Blanco MA. Discovery of insect and human dengue virus host factors. Nature. 2009;**458**:1047-1050. doi:10.1038/nature07967

[52] Duan X, Lu X, Li J, Liu Y. Novel binding between pre-membrane protein and vacuolar ATPase is required for efficient dengue virus secretion. Biochemical and Biophysical Research Communications. 2008;**373**:319-324. doi:10.1016/j.bbrc.2008.06.041

[53] Shapira SD, Gat-Viks I, Shum BO, Dricot A, de Grace MM, Wu L, Gupta PB, Hao T, Silver SJ, Root DE, Hill DE, Regev A, Hacohen N. A physical and regulatory map of host-influenza interactions reveals pathways in H_1N_1 infection. Cell. 2009;**139**:1255-1267. doi:10.1016/j.cell.2009.12.018

[54] Falcon AM, Fortes P, Marion RM, Beloso A, Ortin J. Interaction of influenza virus NS1 protein and the human homologue of Staufen *in vivo* and *in vitro*. Nucleic Acids Research. 1999;**27**:2241-2247.

[55] Gao L, Tu H, Shi ST, Lee KJ, Asanaka M, Hwang SB, Lai MM. Interaction with a ubiquitin-like protein enhances the ubiquitination and degradation of hepatitis C virus RNA-dependent RNA polymerase. Journal of Virology. 2003;**77**:4149-4159.

[56] Taguwa S, Okamoto T, Abe T, Mori Y, Suzuki T, Moriishi K, Matsuura Y. Human butyrate-induced transcript 1 interacts with hepatitis C virus NS5A and regulates viral replication. Journal of Virology. 2008;**82**:2631-2641. doi:10.1128/JVI.02153-07

[57] Ambrosino C, Palmieri C, Puca A, Trimboli F, Schiavone M, Olimpico F, Ruocco MR, di Leva F, Toriello M, Quinto I, Venuta S, Scala G. Physical and functional interaction of HIV-1 Tat with E2F-4, a transcriptional regulator of mammalian cell cycle. Journal of Biological Chemistry. 2002;**277**:31448-31458. doi:10.1074/jbc.M112398200

[58] Kalpana GV, Marmon S, Wang W, Crabtree GR, Goff SP. Binding and stimulation of HIV-1 integrase by a human homolog of yeast transcription factor SNF5. Science. 1994;**266**:2002-2006.

[59] Khadka S, Vangeloff AD, Zhang C, Siddavatam P, Heaton NS, Wang L, Sengupta R, Sahasrabudhe S, Randall G, Gribskov M, Kuhn RJ, Perera R, LaCount DJ. A physical

interaction network of dengue virus and human proteins. Molecular & Cellular Proteomics. 2011;**10**:M111.012187. doi:10.1074/mcp.M111.012187

[60] Le Breton M, Meyniel-Schicklin L, Deloire A, Coutard B, Canard B, de Lamballerie X, Andre P, Rabourdin-Combe C, Lotteau V, Davoust N. Flavivirus NS3 and NS5 proteins interaction network: a high-throughput yeast two-hybrid screen. BMC Microbiology. 2011;**11**:234. doi:10.1186/1471-2180-11-234

[61] Mairiang D, Zhang H, Sodja A, Murali T, Suriyaphol P, Malasit P, Limjindaporn T, Finley RL, Jr. Identification of new protein interactions between dengue fever virus and its hosts, human and mosquito. PLoS One. 2013;**8**:e53535. doi:10.1371/journal.pone.0053535

[62] Sawasaki T, Ogasawara T, Morishita R, Endo Y. A cell-free protein synthesis system for high-throughput proteomics. Proceedings of the National Academy of Sciences of the United States of America. 2002;**99**:14652-14657. doi:10.1073/pnas.232580399

[63] Takahashi H, Takahashi C, Moreland NJ, Chang YT, Sawasaki T, Ryo A, Vasudevan SG, Suzuki Y, Yamamoto N. Establishment of a robust dengue virus NS3-NS5 binding assay for identification of protein-protein interaction inhibitors. Antiviral Research. 2012;**96**:305-314. doi:10.1016/j.antiviral.2012.09.023

[64] Takeda H, Ogasawara T, Ozawa T, Muraguchi A, Jih PJ, Morishita R, Uchigashima M, Watanabe M, Fujimoto T, Iwasaki T, Endo Y, Sawasaki T. Production of monoclonal antibodies against GPCR using cell-free synthesized GPCR antigen and biotinylated liposome-based interaction assay. Scientific Reports. 2015;**5**:11333. doi:10.1038/srep11333

[65] Takahashi H, Uematsu A, Yamanaka S, Imamura M, Nakajima T, Doi K, Yasuoka S, Takahashi C, Takeda H, Sawasaki T. Establishment of a wheat cell-free synthesized protein array containing 250 human and mouse E3 ubiquitin ligases to identify novel interaction between E3 ligases and substrate proteins. PLoS One. 2016;**11**:e0156718. doi:10.1371/journal.pone.0156718

[66] Masaki T, Matsunaga S, Takahashi H, Nakashima K, Kimura Y, Ito M, Matsuda M, Murayama A, Kato T, Hirano H, Endo Y, Lemon SM, Wakita T, Sawasaki T, Suzuki T. Involvement of hepatitis C virus NS5A hyperphosphorylation mediated by casein kinase I-alpha in infectious virus production. Journal of Virology. 2014;**88**:7541-7555. doi:10.1128/JVI.03170-13

[67] Miyakawa K, Sawasaki T, Matsunaga S, Tokarev A, Quinn G, Kimura H, Nomaguchi M, Adachi A, Yamamoto N, Guatelli J, Ryo A. Interferon-induced SCYL2 limits release of HIV-1 by triggering PP2A-mediated dephosphorylation of the viral protein Vpu. Science Signaling 2012;**5**:ra73. doi:10.1126/scisignal.2003212

[68] Kudoh A, Takahama S, Sawasaki T, Ode H, Yokoyama M, Okayama A, Ishikawa A, Miyakawa K, Matsunaga S, Kimura H, Sugiura W, Sato H, Hirano H, Ohno S, Yamamoto N, Ryo A. The phosphorylation of HIV-1 Gag by atypical protein kinase C facilitates viral infectivity by promoting Vpr incorporation into virions. Retrovirology. 2014;**11**:9. doi:10.1186/1742-4690-11-9

[69] Tan BH, Suzuki Y, Takahashi H, Ying PH, Takahashi C, Han Q, Chin WX, Chao SH, Sawasaki T, Yamamoto N, Suzuki Y. Identification of RFPL3 protein as a novel E3 ubiquitin ligase modulating the integration activity of human immunodeficiency virus, type 1 preintegration complex using a microtiter plate-based assay. Journal of Biological Chemistry. 2014;**289**:26368-26382. doi:10.1074/jbc.M114.561662

[70] Matsuoka K, Komori H, Nose M, Endo Y, Sawasaki T. Simple screening method for autoantigen proteins using the N-terminal biotinylated protein library produced by wheat cell-free synthesis. Journal of Proteome Research. 2010;**9**:4264-4273. doi:10.1021/pr9010553

[71] Ullman EF, Kirakossian H, Singh S, Wu ZP, Irvin BR, Pease JS, Switchenko AC, Irvine JD, Dafforn A, Skold CN, et al. Luminescent oxygen channeling immunoassay: measurement of particle binding kinetics by chemiluminescence. Proceedings of the National Academy of Sciences of the United States of America. 1994;**91**:5426-5430.

[72] Matsunaga S, Sawasaki T, Ode H, Morishita R, Furukawa A, Sakuma R, Sugiura W, Sato H, Katahira M, Takaori-Kondo A, Yamamoto N, Ryo A. Molecular and enzymatic characterization of XMRV protease by a cell-free proteolytic analysis. Journal of Proteomics. 2012;**75**:4863-4873. doi:10.1016/j.jprot.2012.05.047

[73] Hershko A, Ciechanover A. The ubiquitin system for protein degradation. Annual Review of Biochemistry. 1992;**61**:761-807. doi:10.1146/annurev.bi.61.070192.003553

[74] Loo YM, Fornek J, Crochet N, Bajwa G, Perwitasari O, Martinez-Sobrido L, Akira S, Gill MA, Garcia-Sastre A, Katze MG, Gale M, Jr. Distinct RIG-I and MDA5 signaling by RNA viruses in innate immunity. Journal of Virology. 2008;**82**:335-345. doi:10.1128/JVI.01080-07

[75] Nasirudeen AM, Wong HH, Thien P, Xu S, Lam KP, Liu DX. RIG-I, MDA5 and TLR3 synergistically play an important role in restriction of dengue virus infection. PLoS Neglected Tropical Diseases. 2011;**5**:e926. doi:10.1371/journal.pntd.0000926

[76] Tsai YT, Chang SY, Lee CN, Kao CL. Human TLR3 recognizes dengue virus and modulates viral replication *in vitro*. Cellular Microbiology. 2009;**11**:604-615. doi:10.1111/j.1462-5822.2008.01277.x

[77] Liang Z, Wu S, Li Y, He L, Wu M, Jiang L, Feng L, Zhang P, Huang X. Activation of toll-like receptor 3 impairs the dengue virus serotype 2 replication through induction of IFN-beta in cultured hepatoma cells. PLoS One. 2011;**6**:e23346. doi:10.1371/journal.pone.0023346

[78] Takeuchi O, Akira S. Pattern recognition receptors and inflammation. Cell. 2010;**140**:805-820. doi:10.1016/j.cell.2010.01.022

[79] Honda K, Takaoka A, Taniguchi T. Type I interferon [corrected] gene induction by the interferon regulatory factor family of transcription factors. Immunity. 2006;**25**:349-360. doi:10.1016/j.immuni.2006.08.009

[80] Schneider WM, Chevillotte MD, Rice CM. Interferon-stimulated genes: a complex web of host defenses. Annual Review of Immunology. 2014;**32**:513-545. doi:10.1146/annurev-immunol-032713-120231

[81] Sen GC. Viruses and interferons. Annual Review of Microbiology. 2001;**55**:255-281. doi:10.1146/annurev.micro.55.1.255

[82] Kane M, Zang TM, Rihn SJ, Zhang F, Kueck T, Alim M, Schoggins J, Rice CM, Wilson SJ, Bieniasz PD. Identification of interferon-stimulated genes with antiretroviral activity. Cell Host Microbe. 2016;**20**:392-405. doi:10.1016/j.chom.2016.08.005

[83] Schoggins JW, Wilson SJ, Panis M, Murphy MY, Jones CT, Bieniasz P, Rice CM. A diverse range of gene products are effectors of the type I interferon antiviral response. Nature. 2011;**472**:481-485. doi:10.1038/nature09907

[84] Brass AL, Huang IC, Benita Y, John SP, Krishnan MN, Feeley EM, Ryan BJ, Weyer JL, van der Weyden L, Fikrig E, Adams DJ, Xavier RJ, Farzan M, Elledge SJ. The IFITM proteins mediate cellular resistance to influenza A H1N1 virus, West Nile virus, and dengue virus. Cell. 2009;**139**:1243-1254. doi:10.1016/j.cell.2009.12.017

[85] Chan YK, Huang IC, Farzan M. IFITM proteins restrict antibody-dependent enhancement of dengue virus infection. PLoS One. 2012;**7**:e34508. doi:10.1371/journal.pone.0034508

[86] Shu Q, Lennemann NJ, Sarkar SN, Sadovsky Y, Coyne CB. ADAP2 is an interferon stimulated gene that restricts RNA virus entry. PLoS Pathogens. 2015;**11**:e1005150. doi:10.1371/journal.ppat.1005150

[87] Jiang D, Weidner JM, Qing M, Pan XB, Guo H, Xu C, Zhang X, Birk A, Chang J, Shi PY, Block TM, Guo JT. Identification of five interferon-induced cellular proteins that inhibit West Nile virus and dengue virus infections. Journal of Virology. 2010;**84**:8332-8341. doi:10.1128/JVI.02199-09

[88] Helbig KJ, Carr JM, Calvert JK, Wati S, Clarke JN, Eyre NS, Narayana SK, Fiches GN, McCartney EM, Beard MR. Viperin is induced following dengue virus type-2 (DENV-2) infection and has anti-viral actions requiring the C-terminal end of viperin. PLoS Neglected Tropical Diseases. 2013;**7**:e2178. doi:10.1371/journal.pntd.0002178

[89] Fink J, Gu F, Ling L, Tolfvenstam T, Olfat F, Chin KC, Aw P, George J, Kuznetsov VA, Schreiber M, Vasudevan SG, Hibberd ML. Host gene expression profiling of dengue virus infection in cell lines and patients. PLoS Neglected Tropical Diseases. 2007;**1**:e86. doi:10.1371/journal.pntd.0000086

[90] Pan XB, Han JC, Cong X, Wei L. BST2/tetherin inhibits dengue virus release from human hepatoma cells. PLoS One. 2012;**7**:e51033. doi:10.1371/journal.pone.0051033

[91] Hishiki T, Han Q, Arimoto K, Shimotohno K, Igarashi T, Vasudevan SG, Suzuki Y, Yamamoto N. Interferon-mediated ISG15 conjugation restricts dengue virus 2 replication. Biochemical and Biophysical Research Communications. 2014;**448**:95-100. doi:10.1016/j.bbrc.2014.04.081

[92] Dai J, Pan W, Wang P. ISG15 facilitates cellular antiviral response to dengue and West Nile virus infection *in vitro*. Virology Journal. 2011;8:468. doi:10.1186/1743-422X-8-468

[93] Schoggins JW, Dorner M, Feulner M, Imanaka N, Murphy MY, Ploss A, Rice CM. Dengue reporter viruses reveal viral dynamics in interferon receptor-deficient mice and sensitivity to interferon effectors *in vitro*. Proceedings of the National Academy of Sciences of the United States of America. 2012;109:14610-14615. doi:10.1073/pnas.1212379109

[94] Yi Z, Sperzel L, Nurnberger C, Bredenbeek PJ, Lubick KJ, Best SM, Stoyanov CT, Law LM, Yuan Z, Rice CM, MacDonald MR. Identification and characterization of the host protein DNAJC14 as a broadly active flavivirus replication modulator. PLoS Pathogens. 2011;7:e1001255. doi:10.1371/journal.ppat.1001255

[95] Suzuki Y, Chin WX, Han Q, Ichiyama K, Lee CH, Eyo ZW, Ebina H, Takahashi H, Takahashi C, Tan BH, Hishiki T, Ohba K, Matsuyama T, Koyanagi Y, Tan YJ, Sawasaki T, Chu JJ, Vasudevan SG, Sano K, Yamamoto N. Characterization of RyDEN (C19orf66) as an interferon-stimulated cellular inhibitor against dengue virus replication. PLoS Pathogens. 2016;12:e1005357. doi:10.1371/journal.ppat.1005357

[96] Diamond MS, Roberts TG, Edgil D, Lu B, Ernst J, Harris E. Modulation of dengue virus infection in human cells by alpha, beta, and gamma interferons. Journal of Virology. 2000;74:4957-4966.

[97] Mangus DA, Evans MC, Jacobson A. Poly(A)-binding proteins: multifunctional scaffolds for the post-transcriptional control of gene expression. Genome Biology. 2003;4:223. doi:10.1186/gb-2003-4-7-223

[98] Wolin SL, Cedervall T. The La protein. Annual Review of Biochemistry. 2002;**71**:375-403. doi:10.1146/annurev.biochem.71.090501.150003

[99] Merret R, Descombin J, Juan YT, Favory JJ, Carpentier MC, Chaparro C, Charng YY, Deragon JM, Bousquet-Antonelli C. XRN4 and LARP1 are required for a heat-triggered mRNA decay pathway involved in plant acclimation and survival during thermal stress. Cell Reports. 2013;**5**:1279-1293. doi:10.1016/j.celrep.2013.11.019

[100] Tcherkezian J, Cargnello M, Romeo Y, Huttlin EL, Lavoie G, Gygi SP, Roux PP. Proteomic analysis of cap-dependent translation identifies LARP1 as a key regulator of 5'TOP mRNA translation. Genes and Development. 2014;**28**:357-371. doi:10.1101/gad.231407.113

[101] Kozlov G, Safaee N, Rosenauer A, Gehring K. Structural basis of binding of P-body-associated proteins GW182 and ataxin-2 by the Mlle domain of poly(A)-binding protein. Journal of Biological Chemistry. 2010;285:13599-13606. doi:10.1074/jbc.M109.089540

[102] Balinsky CA, Schmeisser H, Wells AI, Ganesan S, Jin T, Singh K, Zoon KC. IRAV (FLJ11286), an interferon stimulated gene with antiviral activity against dengue virus, interacts with MOV10. Journal of Virology. 2016. doi:10.1128/JVI.01606-16

[103] Kurane I, Innis BL, Nimmannitya S, Nisalak A, Meager A, Ennis FA. High levels of interferon alpha in the sera of children with dengue virus infection. American Journal of Tropical Medicine and Hygiene. 1993;48:222-229.

[104] Ajariyakhajorn C, Mammen MP, Jr., Endy TP, Gettayacamin M, Nisalak A, Nimmannitya S, Libraty DH. Randomized, placebo-controlled trial of non-pegylated and pegylated forms of recombinant human alpha interferon 2a for suppression of dengue virus viremia in rhesus monkeys. Antimicrobial Agents and Chemotherapy. 2005;49:4508-4514. doi:10.1128/AAC.49.11.4508-4514.2005

[105] Green AM, Beatty PR, Hadjilaou A, Harris E. Innate immunity to dengue virus infection and subversion of antiviral responses. Journal of Molecular Biology. 2014;426:1148-1160. doi:10.1016/j.jmb.2013.11.023

[106] Manokaran G, Finol E, Wang C, Gunaratne J, Bahl J, Ong EZ, Tan HC, Sessions OM, Ward AM, Gubler DJ, Harris E, Garcia-Blanco MA, Ooi EE. Dengue subgenomic RNA binds TRIM25 to inhibit interferon expression for epidemiological fitness. Science. 2015;350:217-221. doi:10.1126/science.aab3369

[107] Bidet K, Dadlani D, Garcia-Blanco MA. G3BP1, G3BP2 and CAPRIN1 are required for translation of interferon stimulated mRNAs and are targeted by a dengue virus non-coding RNA. PLoS Pathogens. 2014;**10**:e1004242. doi:10.1371/journal.ppat.1004242

Chapter 2

Travelling with Dengue: From the Skin to the Nodes

Edith Marcial-Juárez, Juan Carlos Yam-Puc,
Leticia Cedillo-Barrón, Julio García-Cordero,
Juana Calderón-Amador,
Raúl Antonio Maqueda-Alfaro, Karina Ruiz-Tovar,
Nonantzin Beristain-Covarrubias,
Mariana Orozco-Uribe,
Alejandro Escobar-Gutiérrez and
Leopoldo Flores-Romo

Additional information is available at the end of the chapter

http://dx.doi.org/10.5772/intechopen.68338

Abstract

Dengue virus (DENV) infects humans through the skin. The early infection and encounters between DENV and cutaneous immune and non-immune cells only recently are under investigation. We have reported DENV-infected cutaneous dendritic cells (DCs), also keratinocytes and dermal fibroblasts permissive to DENV infection. Now, upon cutaneously inoculating fluorescently labeled DENV into immune-competent mice, we found DENV mostly in dermis from 1 h post-inoculation. Afterwards, DENV rapidly localized in the subcapsular sinus of draining lymph nodes (DLNs) associated with CD169+ macrophages, suggesting virus travelling through lymph flow. However, DENV association with CD11c+ DCs in the paracortex and T:B border suggests DENV being ferried from the skin to DLNs by DCs too. DENV was not associated with F4/80+ macrophages nor with DEC205+ DCs, but it was inside B cell follicles early after cutaneous inoculation. DENV inside B follicles likely affects the development of humoral responses. Antibody responses deserve very careful scrutiny as neutralizing memory antibodies are crucial to counteract homotypic reinfections whereas non-neutralizing ones might facilitate heterotypic DENV infection or even Zika infection, another flavivirus. Unravelling the DENV journey from skin to lymph into regional nodes and the cellular compartments will aid to understand the disease, its pathology and how to counteract it.

Keywords: dengue virus, skin, lymph nodes, immune tissues, macrophages, dendritic cells, B cell follicles

1. Introduction

Dengue virus (DENV) is an important viral pathogen affecting every year almost 400 million people worldwide [1]. Over the past 50 years, the incidence of dengue has increased 30-fold mainly in tropical and subtropical areas causing serious public health problems [2]. DENV triggers a diversity of clinical manifestations, from an asymptomatic infection in the majority of cases, to a mild febrile illness or a life-threatening hemorrhagic disease such as severe dengue (SD) or dengue shock syndrome (DSS) [3].

DENV is transmitted to humans when a priorly infected *Aedes aegypti* female mosquito bites to take a ~4.2 μl blood meal by probing around 141 s in the skin of a healthy person [4, 5]. By the time that half-length (~0.9 mm) of the proboscis is inserted, around 50,000 DENV plaque-forming units are deposited in the dermis, where a variety of resident immune and non-immune cells are located, including dermal dendritic cells (DCs), macrophages (Mfs), T lymphocytes, mast cells, keratinocytes, fibroblasts, etc., as well as lymphatic and blood vessels through which migrating cells travel to lymph nodes (LNs) and arrive at the skin [6–9].

While the regional (cutaneous) responses to DENV entrance are recently under intense scrutiny [10–14], less much is known about how exactly DENV gets its way into lymphatic vessels, secondary lymphoid tissues (if at all) and to which cells might be associated in each of these compartments. By infecting immune-competent mice through the skin, we recently demonstrated not only a strong germinal center (GC) reaction in the draining lymph nodes (DLNs) but also the presence of viral proteins inside these organs [13]. Others have also reported viral proteins inside LNs (NS1, NS3, PrM and E protein) both in humans and mice, suggesting that at least the interactions of viral antigens (Ags) with LN-immune cells are taking place [13, 15, 16].

There is scarce information of the early events happening in the skin during DENV entrance. Some authors have reported an immunomodulatory environment by the mosquito saliva [17, 18], for instance, downregulation of antiviral molecules such as interferon β (IFN-β), IFN-γ, some pattern recognition receptors, or even sustained viremia, among others, helping to establish the infection [19, 20]. It has also been demonstrated a productive infection of fibroblasts, keratinocytes, DCs and Langerhans cells in the skin, but whether these cells participate in the global pathology of the disease remains unclear [10–12, 14, 21].

The appropriate interactions between Ags and immune system cells are essential to start an efficient adaptive immune response in secondary lymphoid tissues such as LNs. For most Ags—including pathogens—it is not well known how exactly they reach LNs and then the subcompartments within, for instance, the B cell follicles. Experimental evidence suggests that certain free Ags could reach LNs directly by lymph flow and then distribute by subcapsular (SCS) and medullary sinus or by means of conduits inside [22–25]. These Ags could also be ferried to nodes by sentinel cells coming from peripheral tissues such as the skin or mucosae. Of note, these various paths of Ag transport are highly dependent on Ag size [22].

However, there is no information on how DENV reaches the DLNs after cutaneous infection, where exactly DENV might be localized inside DLNs (if it does), and whether the first contact between DENV and immune cells could influence subsequent immune responses, for instance, neutralizing or facilitating antibodies.

We aimed at assessing the natural *in vivo* route of DENV, from its entrance through the skin until its arrival and distribution inside regional DLN, as well as, its potential association with antigen presenting cells (APCs).

2. Materials and methods

2.1. Mice

Adult male BALB/c mice were used for all the experiments. Mice were fed *ad libitum* and housed in a specific pathogen-free environment at the local animal facilities, UPEAL. The experimental procedures were approved by the ethical committee of the Center for Advanced Research, The National Polytechnic Institute, Cinvestav-IPN. A group of mice was cutaneously inoculated in the shaved inguinal region with a single dosage of 1×10^6 PFU of fluorescently labeled DENV serotype 2, another group with 5 μg of Alexa Fluor 555-Ovalbumin (Life Technologies; Eugene, OR, USA) and the control group with sterile phosphate-buffered saline (PBS) only. After 1, 3, 6, 12 and 24 hours post-inoculation (hpi), small pieces of skin at the inoculation site and DLNs were extracted and processed either to perform flow cytometry or *in situ* fluorescence, as indicated.

2.2. Antibodies and reagents

The following primary antibodies were used: rat anti-F4/80 (Cl:A3-1), rat anti-CD169 (MOMA-1), both were purchased from Serotec-Bio-Rad (Kidlington, UK); hamster anti-CD11c (HL3), rat anti-B220 (RA3-6B2), rat anti-Gr-1 (RB6-8C5), rat anti-I-A/I-E (2G9), all purchased from BD Pharmingen (San Diego, CA, USA) and rat anti-DEC-205 (205yekta) was purchased from eBioscience (San Diego, CA, USA). Primary antibodies were used directly coupled to allophycocyanin, fluorescein isothiocyanate, PerCP/Cy5.5 or were detected by the following secondary reagents: donkey anti-rat Alexa Fluor 488 purchased from Life Technologies (Eugene, OR, USA) and Cy5-streptavidin and 4′,6-diamino-2-fenilindol (DAPI) purchased from Invitrogen (San Francisco, CA, USA).

2.3. Obtaining dengue virus stock

We obtained DENV stock *in vitro* by infecting the insect cell line C6/36 (from *Aedes albopictus* larvae) with brain extracts of infected neonate mice. C6/36 cells were grown in minimum essential medium eagle (MEM) supplemented with 10% Fetal Bovine Serum (Gibco), Amphotericin B, Penicillin, Streptomycin, Pyruvate, Vitamins and L-glutamine, at 34°C in 75-cm^2 culture flask (Corning). Infection was performed when cells reached 95% confluency. After 48 h post-infection, cell supernatant containing DENV was collected and concentrated with Amicon Centrifugal Filter Units (Merk Millipore, Co. Cork, IRL). Quantification of infectious virions was performed by means of a plaque forming assay in Baby Hamster Kidney cell (BHK-21) and reported as Plaque-Forming Units (PFU)/ml.

2.4. Fluorescent labeling of dengue virus

For *in vivo* DENV tracking in tissues (skin and LNs), we labeled DENV with a strong red fluorescent dye (PKH-26, Sigma). Briefly, DENV was mixed with PKH-26 dye in the appropriate diluent and incubated for 5 min at room temperature. To stop the reaction, we added washing buffer (10% Fetal Bovine Serum in PBS). Because of the virus size, we applied ultrafiltration using centrifugal filter units and centrifuged at 4000 × *g* for 20 min at 4°C. The last step of washing was carried out only with cold sterile PBS.

2.5. Immunofluorescence of LNs and skin

DLN and skin samples were obtained after 1, 3, 6, 12 and 24 hpi from the different groups of experimental animals: PBS-inoculated mice, mice injected with Ovalbumin (OVA) tagged with Alexa Fluor-555 or mice inoculated with fluorescently labeled DENV. Tissues were embedded in optimal cutting temperature (OCT) compound Tissue Tek (Sakura FineTek, Torrance, CA, USA), frozen in liquid nitrogen and cut into 5 μm sections on a cryostat (Leica). Cryosections were put on poly-L-lysine-coated glass slides and fixed with ethanol for 7 min at −20°C. To identify Mfs, we used F4/80 and CD169 antibodies, CD11c and DEC-205 antibodies for DCs and B220 antibody for B lymphocytes; tissue sections were immunolabeled overnight at 4°C with the corresponding primary antibodies. After three washing steps, fluorescent secondary antibodies or streptavidin were incubated during 1 h or 15 min, respectively. Images were scanned with Leica TCS SP8 AOBS Confocal microscopy using objectives with 10× and 40× magnification and analyzed with Leica Software.

2.6. Flow cytometry of lymph node cell suspensions

DLNs were obtained 1, 3, 6, 12 and 24 h after animals were inoculated in the skin with either PBS as a control, or with fluorescently labeled DENV. The cell suspension obtained was blocked with Universal Blocker (BioGenex Laboratories, San Ramón, CA). Then, single-cell suspension was incubated with anti-CD11c, anti-I-A/I-E, anti-Gr-1, anti-F4/80, anti-CD169, anti-B220 and secondary antibodies for 25 min at 4°C in FACS buffer (BSA 1%, NaN_3 0.01% in PBS) to identify APCs and finally fixed with paraformaldehyde 1% for FACS reading. Labeled cell suspensions were acquired with a BD LSR Fortessa III and analyzed with Flowjo X.0.6 for Windows (Ashland, OR).

2.7. Statistical analyses

We performed an ANOVA test for comparing groups using GraphPad Prism v6.0 Software, lines in bars or dots represent ± SEM (standard error of the mean). We considered 95% confidence intervals and significant difference when the P value was <0.05.

3. Results

3.1. Upon cutaneous inoculation DENV is located in the deep dermis and therefore not associated with epidermal DEC-205+ DCs

To assess the distribution of DENV in the skin upon cutaneous (intradermal) inoculation, we used immunocompetent mice and fluorescently labeled DENV. We assessed skin cryosections after 1, 3, 6, 12 and 24 h post-intradermal inoculation of DENV and, as a control we evaluated the distribution of fluorescently labeled OVA at 1 h and 12 hpi. DENV was readily found in the basement of the dermis at all the times evaluated and its presence decreased over time. Putative associations of DENV with epidermal DEC-205+ DCs were not observed, likely because DENV was much deeper than the rather superficial epidermal DEC-205+ cells. At 24 hpi, the skin appears thicker than at early times suggesting recruitment of cells (**Figure 1A**). While no fluorescent signal was detected in skin of mice inoculated only with PBS (**Figure 1A**), fluorescent OVA was clearly seen in the dermis at 1 h but not at 12 hpi (**Figure 1B**).

3.2. Ovalbumin is found in the medullary sinus of the LNs at 1 h but not at 12 h post-cutaneous inoculation

Ovalbumin has been used as model Ag in some experimental approaches to describe the distribution of molecules inside LNs. Because of its molecular size, OVA reaches LNs quickly. We used red fluorescent OVA as a control molecule and evaluated its distribution after 1 h

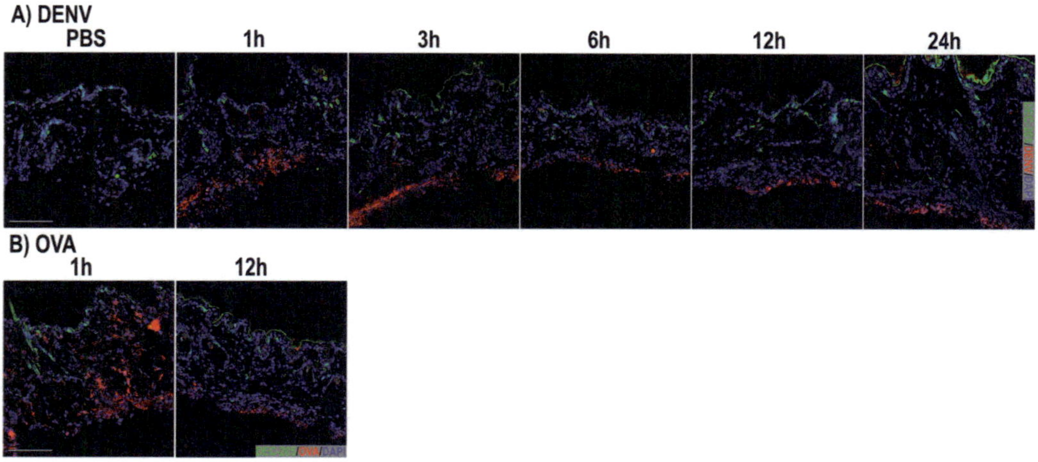

Figure 1. Inoculation of fluorescently labeled DENV allows its identification in the skin of immune-competent mice. Mice were cutaneously inoculated with red fluorescent DENV in the inguinal region and skin cryosections were analyzed after 1, 3, 6, 12 and 24 hpi by confocal microscopy. As controls, mice received either PBS or red fluorescent OVA. DEC-205+ DCs (green) are localized mainly in the epidermal layer in all experimental conditions. (B) Red fluorescent OVA was in the dermis at 1 h but much less was seen at 12 hpi, whereas (A) red fluorescent DENV was located in the deep dermis from 1 hpi decreasing afterwards. In the skin of PBS-inoculated mice, no red fluorescence was detected (left image in (A)). Nuclei were stained with DAPI (blue). Stratum corneum exhibits some autofluorescence at 3 h and 24 hpi (A) and 12 hpi (B). Bar scale = 300 μm. Images are representative of six skin sections per experimental group.

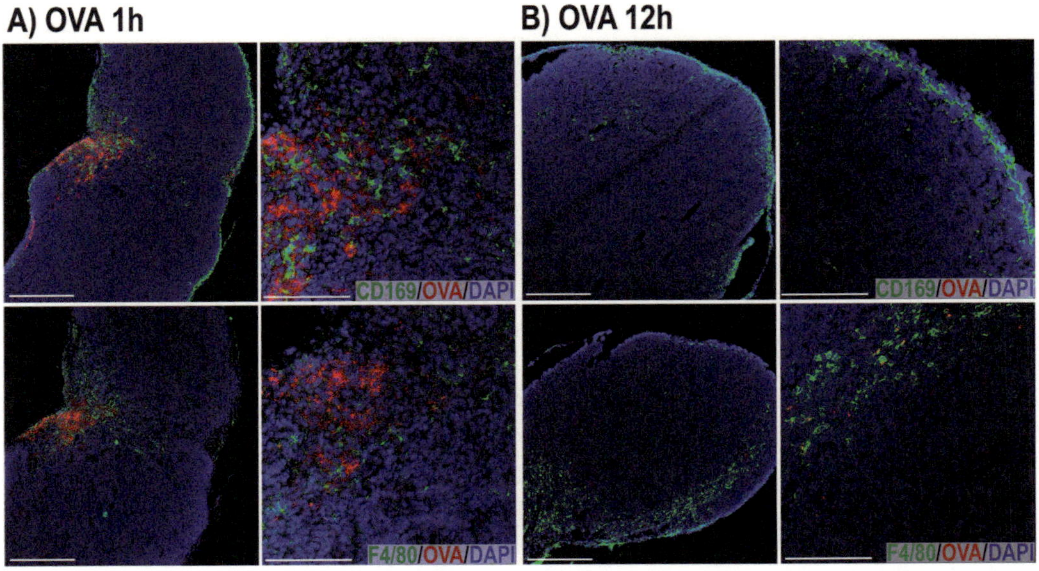

Figure 2. Distribution of red fluorescent OVA in LNs after cutaneous inoculation. DLNs from mice cutaneously inoculated with red fluorescent OVA were harvested at (A) 1 hpi and (B) 12 hpi. CD169+ (top images) and F4/80+ (bottom images) Mfs are seen in green, whereas nuclei are seen in blue. Red fluorescent OVA is clearly observed in the medullary sinus of DLNs at 1 hpi, but not at 12 hpi. The distribution of OVA seems contained by the SCS Mfs but not by F4/80+ Mfs. Bar scale = 300 μm (left images) and 100 μm (right images). Images are representative of six LNs per experimental group.

and 12 hpi. At 1 hpi, OVA was found in the medullary sinus mainly associated with CD169+ Mfs and much less with F4/80+ Mfs (**Figure 2A**). At 12 hpi, only scarce red fluorescence was detected in F4/80+ cells (**Figure 2B**).

3.3. Cutaneous DENV reaches lymph node B follicles since 1 h post-inoculation

To ascertain whether DENV was distributed in B cell follicles at early times post-cutaneous inoculation, we obtained DLNs of mice after 1, 3, 6, 12 and 24 hpi. DLNs cryosections were labeled with B220 antibody to identify B lymphocytes. Red fluorescent DENV was clearly identified in the paracortical areas, the SCS, the medullary sinus and in some B cell follicles (top pictures) at early time points. For a more detailed examination of B cell follicles, we used a higher magnification objective (bottom pictures) showing that at 1 hpi, small clusters of DENV mark were present inside follicles in apparent close association with B cells. At 3 hpi, very few associations were detected in follicles probably because most DENV fluorescence was by then seen at the medullary zone. In contrast, at 6 hpi, we observed some DENV mark inside B cell follicles and even in cells with macrophage-like morphology and the red fluorescence apparently in the cytoplasm. At 12 h and 24 hpi, we did not detect fluorescent DENV signal *in situ* (**Figure 3**).

3.4. Inside lymph nodes DENV appears differentially associated with CD169+ and to F4/80+ macrophages *in situ*

Mfs are crucial for the clearance of pathogens and have been classified according to restricted markers and location inside LNs. Mfs located in the medullary sinus—where highly phagocytic activity is carried out—are called medullary Mfs, whereas those delineating the floor

http://dx.doi.org/10.5772/intechopen.68338

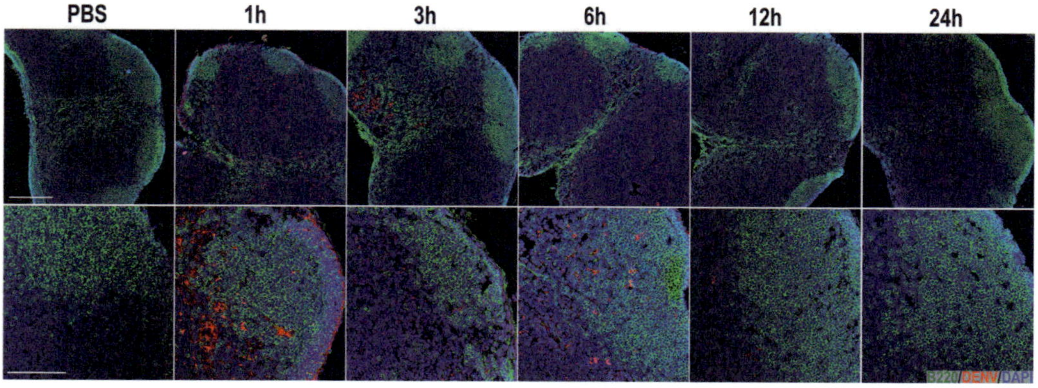

Figure 3. DENV and B cells in DLN cryosections of mice cutaneously inoculated with red fluorescent DENV. LNs cryosections of mice inoculated in the skin with red fluorescent DENV were probed with B220 antibody detected with green fluorescence. Analysis was performed by confocal microscopy at 1, 3, 6, 12 and 24 hpi. We found red fluorescent DENV from 1 h to 6 hpi in B cell follicles (green fluorescence), at 1 hpi DENV was mainly in perifollicular areas. Nuclei were stained with DAPI as observed in blue. As control, DLN sections from PBS-inoculated mice were analyzed, and no red fluorescence was detected (left images). Scale bar = 300 μm (top images) and 100 μm (bottom images). Images are representative of six LNs per experimental group.

of SCS are called SCS Mfs. Medullary Mfs are either CD169+ or F4/80+, whereas SCS Mfs are CD169+ [26].

We assessed *in situ* in DLNs the potential involvement of CD169+ or/and F4/80+ Mfs in capturing DENV after 1, 3, 6, 12 and 24 h post-cutaneous inoculation. Interestingly, since 1 hpi, many CD169+ cells with seemingly cytoplasmic DENV were observed, mainly in SCS and medullary sinus. DENV was also found in paracotical areas in association with CD169- cells (**Figure 4A**). In contrast, at 1 hpi only few F4/80+ medullary Mfs were associated with DENV (**Figure 4B**). After 3 hpi, DENV was mostly restricted to medullary sinus and the CD169+ Mfs (**Figure 4A**). At this time point, DENV was poorly associated with F4/80+ Mfs. Interestingly, many F4/80- cells, most likely CD169+ Mfs, were observed with large amounts of DENV apparently in small phagocytic vesicles, as was observed at high magnification (**Figure 4B**). After 6 hpi, we still detected DENV signal mainly associated with CD169+ Mfs (**Figure 4A**). At the latest times evaluated (12 and 24 hpi), no red fluorescent signal was detected.

3.5. The CD11c+ DCs in regional lymph nodes are DENV+ from early times post-cutaneous inoculation

DCs migrate from peripheral tissues such as the skin (and mucosae) to secondary lymphoid organs like LNs. Because DENV enters through the skin, it is highly likely that skin DCs might participate in delivering DENV into DLNs. We thus probed DLN cryosections with CD11c and DEC-205 antibodies at 1, 3, 6, 12 and 24 h post-cutaneous inoculation of red fluorescent DENV. At 1 hpi, we found DENV in close association with CD11c+ cells but not with DEC-205+ cells in the DLN paracortex. At 3 hpi, we could not find DENV in the paracortex, neither associated with CD11c+ cells nor with DEC-205+ cells; instead, red fluorescent DENV was restricted to medullary areas. At 6 hpi, DENV was associated with some CD11c+ cells, but not with DEC-205+ cells. As mentioned before, DENV was not detected in regional LNs at 12 h nor at 24 hpi (**Figure 5**).

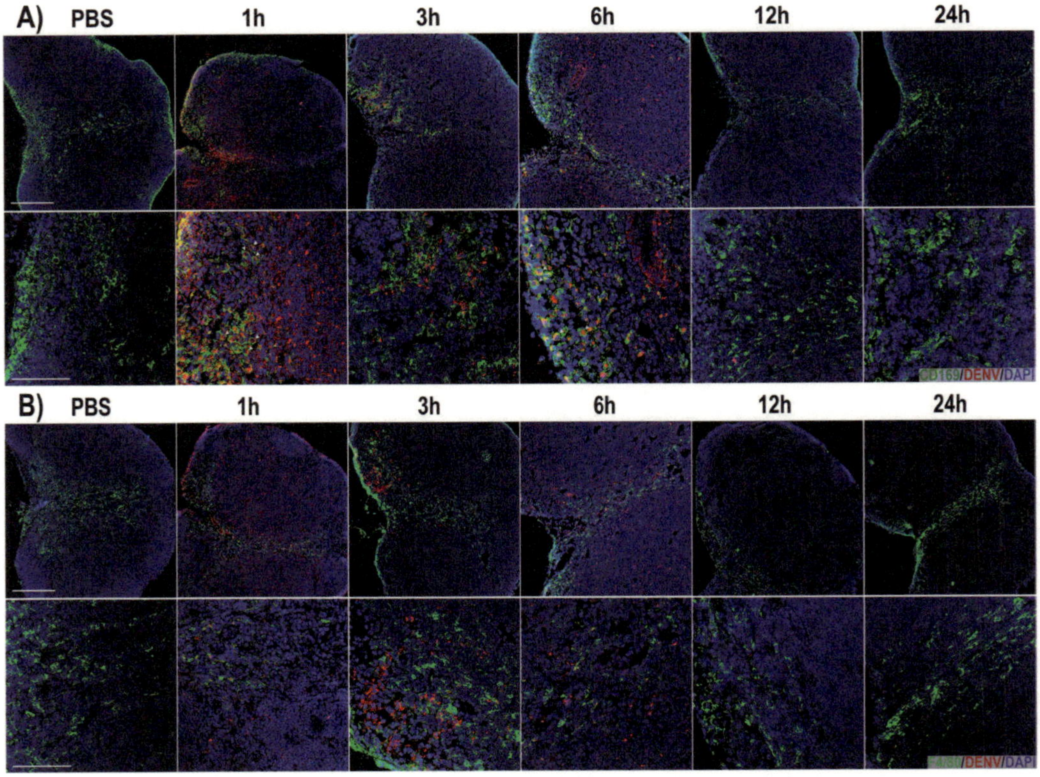

Figure 4. DENV and (CD169+ or F4/80+) macrophages in regional LNs. DLNs from mice inoculated in the skin with PBS or red fluorescent DENV were collected at 1, 3, 6, 12 and 24 hpi, and cryosections were labeled to identify (A) CD169+ or (B) F4/80+ Mfs both in green. Nuclei were stained with DAPI as observed in blue. DLN sections were scanned by confocal microscopy. (A) DENV was distributed in SCS at 1 hpi (yellow color at the edge) and mainly in medullary sinuses apparently in the cytoplasm of CD169+ Mfs from 1 h to 6 hpi (white arrowheads, bottom images). (B) Very few associations of red-fluorescent DENV with F4/80+ Mfs were found in the medullary zones. No red fluorescence was detected in PBS inoculated mice (left images). Bar scale = 300 μm [top images in (A) and (B)] and 100 μm [bottom images in (A) and (B)]. Images are representative of six LNs per experimental group.

3.6. Flow cytometry analysis of Ag presenting cells and DENV in DLNs after cutaneous inoculation

For a more quantitative assessment of APCs associated with DENV, we used DLN cell suspensions from mice inoculated at various times with fluorescent DENV in the skin. A very low proportion (0.06–0.17%) of B cells was positive for DENV at all time points evaluated (1 h-24 hpi). This might be due to the very low number of Ag-specific B cells (**Figure 6A**). CD169+ Mfs were also positive for DENV, with an apparent peak (0.83%) at 3 hpi, which correlates well with the medullary localization observed *in situ* (**Figure 6B**). Regarding F4/80+ Mfs, the proportion of positive cells varied from 0.3 to 0.57% along the experiment, with the maximum at 1 hpi (**Figure 6C**). DCs were identified as Gr-1$^-$, MHC-II$^+$ and CD11c$^+$ cells and were the most abundant DENV+ population. The highest mean proportion (4%) of DENV+

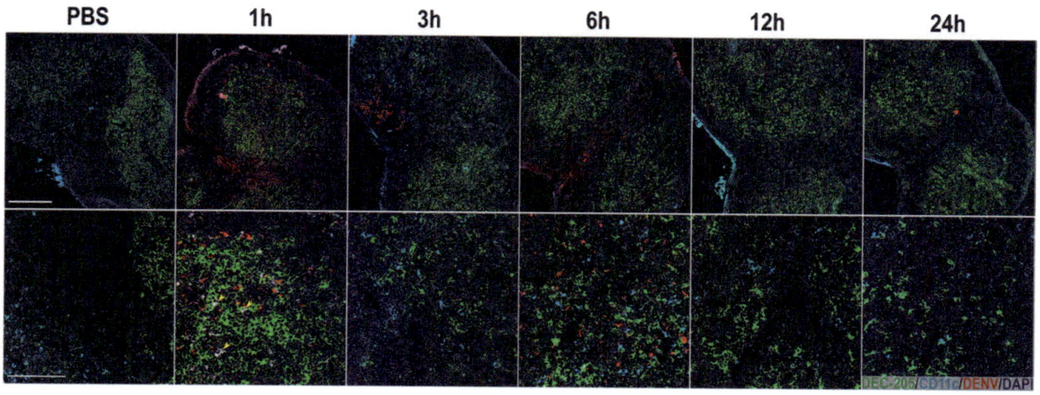

Figure 5. DENV and DCs in regional lymph nodes. Immune-competent mice were intradermally inoculated with red fluorescent DENV, and DLNs were harvested at 1, 3, 6, 12 and 24 hpi. CD11c+ DCs were identified in light blue fluorescence, DEC-205+ DCs in green, whereas nuclei are seen in dark blue. As described, DENV was detected from 1 h to 6 hpi. At 1 hpi, red fluorescent DENV was located in the paracortical area and clearly associated with light blue CD11c+ DCs which then appear white due to merged colors (bottom image, yellow arrowheads indicate white color DCs). Red DENV was not associated with green DEC-205+ DCs. Cryosections of PBS inoculated mice did not show red fluorescence (left images). Bar scale = 300 μm (top images) and 100 μm (bottom images). Images are representative of six LNs per experimental group.

DCs was seen at 1 hpi decreasing afterwards to a minimum (0.85%) at 24 hpi (**Figure 6D**). We integrated all values in a graph (**Figure 6E**) to compare the percentages of all DENV+ APCs assessed. It seems that DCs are the main DENV+ cells, especially at early times post-inoculation, suggesting that either these cells are carrying DENV from skin to the nodes or are the main cells capturing the virus once DENV arrives into the nodes.

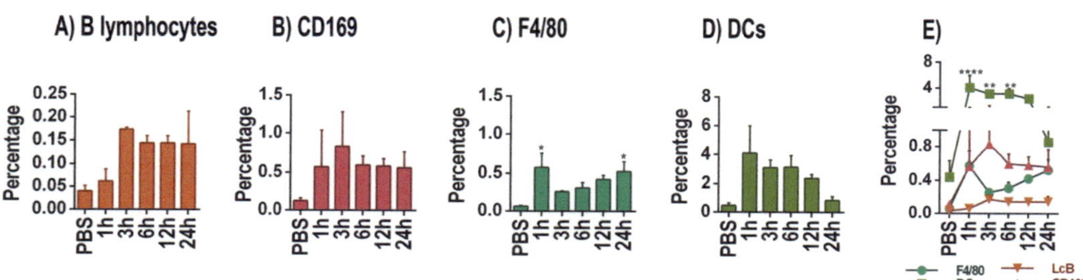

Figure 6. Flow cytometry assessment of DENV+ cells in regional LNs. Cell suspensions of DLNs harvested 1, 3, 6, 12 and 24 h after inoculating red fluorescent DENV were labeled for B cells (B220), Mfs (CD169 and F4/80) and DCs (CD11c). Red fluorescence co-staining was used to determine the percentage of each DENV+ cell population. (A) A very low proportion of DENV+ B cells was observed from 1 h to 24 hpi. (B) The amount of DENV+ CD169+ Mfs was higher than (C) DENV+ F4/80+ Mfs from 1 h to 24 hpi. (D) The proportion of DENV+ CD11c+ DCs was higher than the other populations, reaching a maximum at 1 hpi declining afterwards. Graph in (E) shows the integrated results of all cell subsets during the kinetic follow up. Bars in graphs represent the median ± SEM of percentages, and ANOVA analysis was performed, considering $^{*}p > 0.05$, $^{**}p > 0.01$ and $^{****}p > 0.0001$.

4. Discussion

While many cells in the skin can make contact with DENV during mosquito biting (a topic under intense investigation recently), very few cells will have the ability to capture DENV and to ferry it into lymphatic vessels and from there to secondary lymphoid tissues. Cutaneous DCs can uptake DENV and migrate into DLNs to the DC area, where the most likely cells to make the first immune contacts with DENV+ DCs will be T lymphocytes [27]. Some B cells could also interact with DENV Ags in this area and follow either an extrafollicular response or get into a GC reaction [28, 29]. Still another possibility inside LNs is the display of DENV Ags by Mfs, either in the SCS or deeper in the paracortical and medullary zones [30]. Thus, LNs are crucial organs to establish effective adaptive immune responses. For this, the efficient interaction between immune cells and Ags is needed. The ensuing events upon arrival of Ags inside LNs might depend on how these Ags are getting there, whether the Ag is arriving alone through the lymph flow or is carried by different cells which could be important to the type of the immune response that follows. Herein, we discuss some of these possibilities regarding DENV infection *in vivo*.

DENV enters the human host through the skin while mosquitoes feed. After locating a suitable host, an infected mosquito probes throughout the dermis introducing the proboscis and is during this process that the salivary glands release the virus [31]. Conceivably, viral particles are likely to interact first with the various cells of epidermal and dermal layers. However, both the very early stages of DENV infection and the initial local encounters between DENV and elements of the local immune system *in situ* remain largely unexplored.

By infecting *ex vivo* healthy human skin explants from non-cadaveric samples, our group demonstrated DENV-infected cutaneous DCs [11]. We have also identified that human keratinocytes and dermal fibroblasts are permissive to DENV infection and that they respond by secreting a wide variety of soluble mediators that contribute to induce an immune-activated microenvironment and an antiviral state [10, 11, 32]. Now, upon cutaneous inoculation of fluorescently labeled DENV into immune-competent mice, we evaluated the presence of DENV as well as its localization in both the skin and the DLNs. We did a kinetic follow-up by *in situ* immunofluorescence as well as in cell suspensions by FACS. In the skin, we found the virus localized mostly through the dermis at 1 h post-inoculation, afterwards DENV was distributed deep in the skin. To the best of our knowledge, this is the first time that fluorescently labeled DENV is used to assess its distribution *in vivo*.

Some reports in humans and mice have shown DENV proteins inside LNs, both at the periphery and inside B cell follicles [13, 16, 33–35]. Where the virus is located inside DLNs could influence the first contact with cells from the immune system and the subsequent immune response. However, how DENV reaches the DLNs after cutaneous infection has not been explored *in vivo*. Using the vesicular stomatitis virus, researchers have investigated how viral particles that enter through peripheral tissues are handled within DLNs, identifying a population of Mfs on the floor of the SCS and in the medulla of LNs that capture viral particles within minutes after subcutaneous injection [30]. Similar to other Ags delivered through the skin, the Bluetongue Virus is transported rapidly through the lymph to the DLNs in its natural host the sheep [36].

After 1 h of skin inoculation and once in DLNs, we found DENV associated with CD169+ Mfs from the subcapsular and medullary sinus and with CD11c+ DCs in the paracortical area. The association with these two cell types was seen especially at early times (1–6 h) after cutaneous inoculation. The rapid localization of DENV in the SCS of the DLNs is consistent with delivery of putative cell-free virus through the lymphatic fluid, besides that DCs might be also carrying the virus [36]. In the immune-deficient murine model (AG129 mice), it has been shown that Mfs from the SCS are important controlling the spreading of DENV. These SCS Mfs contained NS1 protein, likely implying that they are trapping DENV Ags or are being actually infected [37]. In these same immune-deficient mice, after intra-footpad inoculation, it was shown that DENV initially targets Mfs of the DLN [38]. As SIGN-R1, the murine homolog of human DC-SIGN is highly expressed on SCS Mfs [39], it is likely that DENV is infecting these Mfs in the DLN. Indeed, DC-SIGN is one of the molecules used by DENV to enter host cells [40].

After the SCS Mfs trap DENV, these cells could translocate surface-bound viral particles across the SCS floor and make DENV Ags available to other cells, for instance, migrating B cells in the underlying follicles. It seems that these Mfs from the SCS act as vigilants against many different pathogens and are able to discriminate between lymph-borne viruses and other particles of similar size [30]. CD169+ Mfs in LNs could capture lymph-borne viruses preventing their systemic dissemination and could guide captured virions across the SCS floor for the efficient activation of follicular B cells [30, 37].

In addition to this, DENV associated with DCs highly likely implies that DENV is transported from the skin to the DLNs by DCs. We and others have found DENV-infected cutaneous DCs in human cadaveric and non-cadaveric healthy skin explants infected *ex vivo* [11, 14, 21]. Thus, DENV might be reaching DLNs also through cutaneous DCs. Also, migratory DENV-infected DCs have been found in the skin DLNs of mice lacking IFN-α/β receptor (IFNAR$^{-/-}$ mice) infected through the skin, suggesting that dermal DCs might be ferrying DENV to regional nodes and likely triggering the adaptive immune response [14].

DCs are specialized sentinel cells that uptake Ags at peripheral tissues and travel to DLNs ferrying Ags to paracortical areas, where B cells migrating toward follicles are likely to encounter these Ags [23, 27, 41]. A hallmark of specific B lymphocyte activation is BCR-mediated capturing/acquisition of Ags. This will facilitate the subsequent Ag presentation from B cells to T cells in order to develop efficient T cell-dependent antibody responses [42]. DCs may provide B cells with broader access to Ags, particularly those of large sizes or associated with particulate materials. Lastly, through Ag presentation to T cells, DCs could subserve functions such as cellular platforms facilitating activation, colocalization and mutual communication of rare Ag-specific T and B cells, whose interaction may ultimately lead to optimal T and B cell responses [41].

Tracking *in vivo* fluorescently labeled DENV from the skin permitted us to know the rapid (1 hpi) localization of DENV in subcapsular and medullary Mfs of DLNs, its association with CD11c+ DCs in the T:B border and the presence of DENV inside B cell follicles. All these events make highly plausible that Ag-specific B cells would be recognizing DENV and makes feasible that they would be receiving T cell help, these cellular interactions are needed to lead to full antibody responses. To this respect, it is worth mentioning that antibody responses to DENV need very careful examination; ideally, these responses should be neutralizing [43, 44]. However, the potentially detrimental impact of non-neutralizing antibodies enhancing the infection *in vivo* is only beginning to be elucidated, not only in heterotypic reinfections with DENV but also in infections with other flaviviruses such as Zika [44–48].

Altogether, these data suggest that after being inoculated into skin, DENV is reaching the regional lymph nodes in at least two ways, through the lymph fluids but also being carried by cells. Travelling with DENV from the skin to the regional LNs will allow us to better understand how the immune system is being alerted or affected and which might be the cells responding at each stage. We believe that it is important to decipher the *in vivo* biology of these cellular responses to DENV entrance, not only for making better models to study early interactions among DENV, skin-resident and LN cells but also to better understand the pathology of DENV.

Acknowledgements

Leticia Cedillo-Barrón, Alejandro Escobar-Gutiérrez, Julio García-Cordero and Leopoldo Flores-Romo are members of the National System of Researchers (SNI) from Mexico. Support from the National Council for Science and Technology (Conacyt) of Mexico was given through the projects 221102 to LF-R and 139542 to AE-G and grant 233347 from Fonsalud to LC-B. Edith Marcial-Juárez, Juan Carlos Yam-Puc, Raúl Antonio Maqueda-Alfaro, Mariana Orozco-Uribe and Nonantzin Beristain-Covarrubias are fellow-holders from Conacyt. The authors acknowledge the invaluable help from Jaime Escobar at the Confocal Microscopy facilities, from Victor Rosales at the FACS facilities and the personnel from the Cinvestav animal facilities (UPEAL), René Pánfilo-Morales, Ricardo Gaxiola-Centeno and Rafael Leyva-Muñoz. The authors also thank Yolanda Sánchez-Chávez for the excellent technical assistance provided.

Author details

Edith Marcial-Juárez[1], Juan Carlos Yam-Puc[1], Leticia Cedillo-Barrón[2], Julio García-Cordero[2], Juana Calderón-Amador[1], Raúl Antonio Maqueda-Alfaro[1], Karina Ruiz-Tovar[3], Nonantzin Beristain-Covarrubias[2], Mariana Orozco-Uribe[1], Alejandro Escobar-Gutiérrez[3] and Leopoldo Flores-Romo[1]*

*Address all correspondence to: lefloresromo@gmail.com

1 Department of Cell Biology, Center for Advanced Research, The National Polytechnic Institute, Cinvestav-IPN, Mexico City, Mexico

2 Department of Molecular Biomedicine, Center for Advanced Research, The National Polytechnic Institute, Cinvestav-IPN, Mexico City, Mexico

3 Department for Immunological Investigations, Institute for Epidemiological Diagnosis and Reference, Health Secretariat, Mexico City, Mexico

References

[1] Bhatt S, Gething PW, Brady OJ, et al. The global distribution and burden of dengue. Nature. 2013;**496**:504-507

[2] World Health Organization (WHO). Global Strategy for Dengue Prevention and Control, 2012-2020. Geneva: WHO Press; 2012

[3] Screaton G, Mongkolsapaya J, Yacoub S, et al. New insights into the immunopathology and control of dengue virus infection. Nature Reviews Immunology. 2015;**15**:745-759

[4] Neville Clements A. The Physiology of Mosquitoes. Pergamon Press. 1963

[5] Daniel TL, Kingsolver JG. Feeding strategy and the mechanics of blood sucking in insects. Journal of Theoretical Biology. 1983;**105**:661-677

[6] Ramasubramanian MK, Barham OM, Swaminathan V. Mechanics of a mosquito bite with applications to microneedle design. Bioinspiration & Biomimetics. 2008;**3**:46001

[7] Styer LM, Kent KA, Albright RG, et al. Mosquitoes inoculate high doses of west nile virus as they probe and feed on live hosts. PLOS Pathogens. 2007;**3**:e132

[8] Fehres CM, Garcia-Vallejo JJ, Unger WWJ, et al. skin-resident antigen-presenting cells: instruction manual for vaccine development. Frontiers in Immunology. 2013;**4**:157

[9] Pasparakis M, Haase I, Nestle FO. Mechanisms regulating skin immunity and inflammation. Nature Reviews Immunology. 2014;**14**:289-301

[10] Bustos-Arriaga J, García-Machorro J, León-Juárez M, et al. Activation of the innate immune response against DENV in normal non-transformed human fibroblasts. PLOS Neglected Tropical Diseases. 2011;**5**:e1420

[11] Limon-Flores AY, Perez-Tapia M, Estrada-Garcia I, et al. Dengue virus inoculation to human skin explants: an effective approach to assess in situ the early infection and the effects on cutaneous dendritic cells. International Journal of Experimental Pathology. 2005;**86**:323-334

[12] David MS, Dimelza SP, Porfirio ND, et al. Innate immune responses in ex vivo skin explants infected with dengue virus. Front in Immunology. 2015;**6**:*Conference Abstract: IMMUNOCOLOMBIA2015-11th Congress of the Latin American Association of Immunology - 10o. Congreso de la Asociación Colombiana de Alergia, Asma e Inmunología.*

[13] Yam-Puc JC, García-Cordero J, Calderón-Amador J, et al. Germinal center reaction following cutaneous dengue virus infection in immune-competent mice. Front in Immunology. 2015;**6**:1-9

[14] Cerny D, Haniffa M, Shin A, et al. Selective susceptibility of human skin antigen presenting cells to productive dengue virus infection. PLOS Pathogens. 2014;**10**:e1004548

[15] Balsitis SJ, Coloma J, Castro G, et al. Tropism of dengue virus in mice and humans defined by viral nonstructural protein 3-specific immunostaining. The American Journal of Tropical Medicine and Hygiene. 2009;**80**:416-424

[16] Bhoopat L, Bhamarapravati N, Attasiri C, et al. Immunohistochemical characterization of a new monoclonal antibody reactive with dengue virus-infected cells in frozen tissue using immunoperoxidase technique. Asian Pacific Journal of Allergy and Immunology. 1996;**14**:107-13

[17] Mores CN, Christofferson RC, Davidson SA. The Role of the mosquito in a dengue human infection model. The Journal of Infectious Diseases. 2014;**209**:S71–S78

[18] Schneider BS, Higgs S. The enhancement of arbovirus transmission and disease by mosquito saliva is associated with modulation of the host immune response. Transactions of the Royal Society of Tropical Medicine and Hygiene. 2008;**102**:400-408

[19] Cox J, Mota J, Sukupolvi-Petty S, et al. Mosquito bite delivery of dengue virus enhances immunogenicity and pathogenesis in humanized mice. Journal of Virology. 2012;**86**:7637-7649

[20] McCracken MK, Christofferson RC, Chisenhall DM, et al. Analysis of early dengue virus infection in mice as modulated by *Aedes aegypti* probing. Journal of Virology. 2014;**88**:1881-9

[21] Wu S-JJ, Grouard-Vogel G, Sun W, et al. Human skin Langerhans cells are targets of dengue virus infection. Nature Medicine. 2000;**6**:816-20

[22] Gretz JE, Norbury CC, Anderson AO, et al. Lymph-borne chemokines and other low molecular weight molecules reach high endothelial venules via specialized conduits while a functional barrier limits access to the lymphocyte microenvironments in lymph node cortex. The Journal of Experimental Medicine. 2000;**192**:1425-1440

[23] Cyster JG. B cell follicles and antigen encounters of the third kind. Nature Immunology. 2010;**11**:989-996

[24] Batista FD, Harwood NE. The who, how and where of antigen presentation to B cells. Nature Reviews Immunology. 2009;**9**:15-27

[25] Carrasco YR, Batista FD. B Cells acquire particulate antigen in a macrophage-rich area at the boundary between the follicle and the subcapsular sinus of the lymph node. Immunity. 2007;**27**:160-171

[26] Gray EE, Cyster JG. Lymph node macrophages. Journal of Innate Immunity. 2012;**4**:424-436

[27] Steinman RM, Pack M, Inaba K. Dendritic cells in the T-cell areas of lymphoid organs. Immunological Reviews. 1997;**156**:25-37

[28] MacLennan ICM. Germinal centers. Annual Review of Immunology. 1994;**12**:117-139

[29] MacLennan ICM, Toellner K-M, Cunningham AF, et al. Extrafollicular antibody responses. *Immunological Reviews.* 2003;**194**:8-18

[30] Junt T, Moseman EA, Iannacone M, et al. Subcapsular sinus macrophages in lymph nodes clear lymph-borne viruses and present them to antiviral B cells. Nature. 2007;**450**:110-114

[31] Platt KB, Linthicum KJ, Myint KS, et al. Impact of dengue virus infection on feeding behavior of *Aedes aegypti*. The American Journal of Tropical Medicine and Hygiene. 1997;**57**:119-25

[32] Bustos-Arriaga J, Mita-Mendoza NK, Lopez-Gonzalez M, et al. Soluble mediators produced by the crosstalk between microvascular endothelial cells and dengue-infected primary dermal fibroblasts inhibit dengue virus replication and increase leukocyte transmigration. Immunologic Research. 2016;**64**:392-403

[33] Aye KS, Charngkaew K, Win N, et al. Pathologic highlights of dengue hemorrhagic fever in 13 autopsy cases from Myanmar. Human Pathology. 2014;**45**:1221-1233

[34] Boonpucknavig S, Vuttiviroj O, Boonpucknavig V. Infection of young adult mice with dengue virus type 2. Transactions of the Royal Society of Tropical Medicine and Hygiene. 1981;**75**:647-653

[35] Jessie K, Fong MY, Devi S, et al. Localization of dengue virus in naturally infected human tissues, by immunohistochemistry and in situ hybridization. The Journal of Infectious Diseases. 2004;**189**:1411-1418

[36] Melzi E, Caporale M, Rocchi M, et al. Follicular dendritic cell disruption as a novel mechanism of virus-induced immunosuppression. Proceedings of the National Academy of Sciences. 2016;**113**:E6238–E6247

[37] Fink K, Ng C, Nkenfou C, et al. Depletion of macrophages in mice results in higher dengue virus titers and highlights the role of macrophages for virus control. European Journal of Immunology. 2009;**39**:2809-2821

[38] Prestwood TR, May MM, Plummer EM, et al. Trafficking and replication patterns reveal splenic macrophages as major targets of dengue virus in mice. Journal of Virology. 2012;**86**:12138-12147

[39] Geijtenbeek TBH. Marginal zone macrophages express a murine homologue of DC-SIGN that captures blood-borne antigens in vivo. Blood. 2002;**100**:2908-2916

[40] Cruz-Oliveira C, Freire JM, Conceicao TM, et al. Receptors and routes of dengue virus entry into the host cells. FEMS Microbiology Reviews. 2015;**39**:155-170

[41] Qi H. Extrafollicular activation of lymph node B cells by antigen-bearing dendritic cells. Science. 2006;**312**:1672-1676

[42] MacLennan ICM, Gulbranson-Judge A, Toellner K-M, et al. The changing preference of T and B cells for partners as T-dependent antibody responses develop. Immunological Reviews. 1997;**156**:53-66

[43] Cedillo-Barrón L, García-Cordero J, Bustos-Arriaga J, et al. Antibody response to dengue virus. Microbes and Infection. 2014;**16**:711-720

[44] Yam-Puc JC, Cedillo-Barrón L, Aguilar-Medina EM, et al. The cellular bases of antibody responses during dengue virus infection. Front in Immunology. 2016;**7**:1-12

[45] Dejnirattisai W, Jumnainsong A, Onsirisakul N, et al. Cross-reacting antibodies enhance dengue virus infection in humans. Science. 2010;**328**:745-748

[46] Dejnirattisai W, Supasa P, Wongwiwat W, et al. Dengue virus sero-cross-reactivity drives antibody-dependent enhancement of infection with zika virus. Nature Immunology. 2016;**17**:1102-1108

[47] Beltramello M, Williams KL, Simmons CP, et al. The human immune response to dengue virus is dominated by highly cross-reactive antibodies endowed with neutralizing and enhancing activity. Cell Host and Microbe. 2010;**8**:271-283

[48] Paul LM, Carlin ER, Jenkins MM, et al. Dengue virus antibodies enhance Zika virus infection. Clinical and Translational Immunology. 2016;**5**:e117

Chapter 3

Assessment of Dengue Fever Severity Through Liver Function Test

Ambreen Zubair, Asim Ahmad Qureshi and
Syed Ahmed Murtaza Jafri

Additional information is available at the end of the chapter

http://dx.doi.org/10.5772/intechopen.68949

Abstract

Objective: To assess the utility of liver function tests (LFTs) for early recognition and prediction of severity of dengue fever in hospitalized patients. *Study Design*: An analytical study. *Place and duration of study:* Services Institute of Medical Science and Fatima Memorial Hospital, Lahore, from September to December 2010. *Methodology*: Admitted cases of dengue fever were divided into three groups: mild, moderate, and severe increases in aminotransferases. Elevation in LFTs was co-related with good or bad outcome i.e. (survival or complication free stay) or (death or complications). Results were analyzed in SPSS version 18. *Results*: Out of the 353 patients with mean age of 37.12 ± 15.45 years, 245 (69.4%) were males and 108 (30.6%) were females. Seventy five patients (21.2%) had mild elevation of aminotransferases (twofold increases), 265 patients (75.1%) had moderate increases (three to fourfold), and 13 (3.7%) had severe (>4 fold increase). Alanine transaminase (ALT) was statistically higher in patients with septicemia, hepatic, and renal failure (p-value ≤0.05). Aspartate transaminase (AST) was higher in almost all complications. Prolonged hospital stay was associated with raised LFTs and greater complications and mortality. AST was found to be twice as much raised as ALT. *Conclusion*: AST and ALT were statistically higher in patients with worse outcome thus can lead to early recognition of high risk cases.

Keywords: dengue fever, liver disease, liver function tests, severity

1. Definition of subject area

Dengue fever has emerged as a biggest global **pandemic** caused by a flavivirus with significant impact on the disease burden in population living in tropical countries with 1–2 epidemics every year [1].

1.1. Dengue virus

Dengue virus (DENV) has **four** serotypes (DEN 1–4). Currently, all the serotypes have diffused in tropical and subtropical regions of the world [2].

1.2. Mode of transmission

DENVs are transmitted via the female mosquito species **Aedes** *Aegypti* and less commonly by *Aedes Albopictus* [2].

1.3. Incubation period

Dengue virus has an incubation period of **3–10** days with average of 5–6 days [3].

1.4. Period of infectivity

Within first 5 days of illness, if Aedes mosquito feeds on patient blood, it will become infective [3].

1.5. Outcome of dengue infection

Majority of dengue infections are **asymptomatic**. Among symptomatic presentation is highly variable from mild **flu**-like illness to classical dengue fever (**DF**) (**bone-break** fever) and even some complicate into dengue hemorrhagic fever (**DHF**) and dengue shock syndrome (**DSS**), which are life threatening (**Table 1**) [4].

If total score >6, then patient has high chances of having dengue fever

- This scoring system carries
- *sensitivity = 90.7%*
- *specificity = 86.9%*
- *positive predictive value = 81.4%*
- *negative predictive value = 93.6%.*
- Chang et al. [5].

2. Description of study

Involvement of liver with deranged liver function tests (LFTs) is likely with dengue fever and which may include mildly raised in serum total bilirubin, increased alanine transaminase (ALT) and aspartate transaminase (**AST**), and decreased in serum albumin which can be a used as a prognostic indicator [6].

1	**Epidemiology**	**Score**
	Recent travel to Southeast Asia or four endemic dengue fever in Taiwan within 1 week	4
2	**Clinical symptom**	
	Skin rash	3
	Bleeding signs (Included petechia, gum bleeding, epistaxis, gastrointestinal bleeding, hemoptysis, hematuria, and menorrhagia)	3
	Fever	2
	Headache, retrobulbar pain, bone pain, myalgia	1
	GI symptoms (poor appetite, abdominal pain, diarrhea and nausea)	1
	Absence of cough and rhinorrhea	1
3	**Differential diagnosis**	
	Fever > 7 days	−8
	Identified infection focus (e.g., Eschar of scrub typhus and upper respiratory infection)	−10

Table 1. Diagnostic criteria for dengue fever.

3. Objectives of the study

The objectives of the chapter are as follows:

1. To evaluate such alterations in the liver function test as an early marker for severity and timely diagnosis of dengue fever complications and severity [7].
2. To identify patients who might develop severe complications.
3. To decrease the degree of in hospital stay by categorizing patients into mild, moderate, and high risk groups according to their raised transaminases (ALT and AST) levels [8].

4. Materials and methods

A study was conducted in different government as well as private tertiary care setups in Lahore from September 2010 to December 2010. The total 353 patients were included in the study. It was a simple **randomized** sample and the study design was a cross-sectional observational study.

4.1. Categorization of patients

Patients were divided into three groups and categorized to have mild, moderate, or severe liver dysfunction. Group I included patients who had twofold or lesser increase in liver enzymes; in group II patients, liver function tests were between twofold and fourfold greater than normal; group III patients had liver function tests greater than fourfold above normal. The correlation of these groups with the development of complications, mortality, and number of days of hospital stay was studied. Good outcome was taken as survival and complication free pattern of disease, while bad outcome was taken as development of complication or mortality.

4.2. Results and conclusion

- The effects of dengue fever on liver are usually asymptomatic but can be atypical and have varied severity. From asymptomatic elevated transaminase levels to fulminant hepatic failure, the variable manifestations are a big challenge to the clinicians treating the condition (**Tables 2–4**).

Variables	Mean	Std. deviation	Minimum	Maximum
Age (years)	37.12	15.456	4	80
Duration of fever	5.49	2.64	1	35

Table 2. Descriptive statistics of demographical variables.

Complications	Severity of disease			Total n = 85
	Mild n = 27	Moderate n = 38	Severe n = 20	
DHF	12 (14. 11%)	11 (12.94%)	1 (1.17%)	24 (28.23%)
DSS	4 (4.7%)	4 (4.7%)	4 (4.7%)	12 (14.11%)
Hemorrhage	8 (9.41%)	18 (21.17%)	3 (3.52%)	29 (34.11%)
Septicemia	0 (0%)	2 (2.35%)	3 (3.52%)	5 (5.88%)
Hepatic failure	0 (0%)	1 (1.17%)	4 (4.7%)	5 (5.88%)
Encephalopathy	2 (2.35%)	1 (1.17%)	1 (1.17%)	4 (4.70%)
Respiratory failure	1 (1.17%)	1 (1.17%)	2 (2.35%)	4 (4.70%)
Renal failure	0 (0%)	0 (0%)	2 (2.35%)	2 (2.35%)
Total	27 (31.76%)	38 (44.70%)	20 (23.52%)	85

Table 3. Complications versus severity of disease.

The reversal of alanine transaminase and aspartate transaminase (ALT to AST) ratio observed in dengue fever as compared to that seen in other viral hepatitis can lead to an early diagnosis of these patients.

- Increasing trend in aminotransferases is associated with major complications and a bad outcome as compared to patients with mild or moderate hepatic dysfunction.
- Severe hepatitis and specifically raised alanine transaminase (ALT) levels are a poor prognostic indicator of outcome in dengue fever.

- The younger age group of patients was directly associated with severely raised levels of alanine transaminase (ALT) and thus contributing to a higher mortality.

4.3. Pathogenesis of DF, DHF, and DSS

Dengue virus presumably affects the reticulo-endothelial system of the body in skin, lymph nodes, spleen, marrow and liver [9].

DHF and DSS are caused by disorder of the immune system. In recovery phase (days 7–14) of first infection, another serotype is superinfected. Then antibodies against first serotype binds with new entrant serotype antigen leading to immune complex formation, their deposition on endothelium leading to widespread vessel wall injury, hemorrhages, and third spacing of fluid [4].

4.4. Dengue virus and liver

The dengue virus affects the liver but mostly, liver involvement is usually subclinical. But it can still lead to acute fulminant hepatic failure in dengue-affected countries. Dengue should be a differential in management of acute fulminant hepatic failure and as a triggering factor in patient with acute on chronic liver failure [6].

Despite being asymptomatic in majority of cases, clinical presentation like acute hepatitis and even acute fulminant liver failure may rarely appear as a complication.

4.5. Pathogenesis of liver injury

Hepatic dysfunction is a crucial feature seen in DENV infection. Hepatocytes and Kupffer cells are prime targets for DENV infection. Pathogenesis of hepatic injury in dengue is believed to be primarily a T cell-mediated process involving interaction between antibodies and the endothelium and a concomitant cytokine storm [7, 10].

4.6. Liver morphology

Liver biopsy and microscopy reveals fatty change (microvesicular) along with hepatocyte necrosis and hyperplasia. Additionally, there is mononuclear cell infiltration at the portal tract along with destruction of Kupffer cells and Councilman bodies [11].

Tests result	Mean	Std. deviation	Minimum	Maximum
TLC	4.7711	2.17496	1	20
ALT	100.29	102.14	11	1102
AST	234.17	136.09	21	1680
PT	16.71	3.59	10	60
APTT	34.40	1.650	19	50

Table 4. Descriptive statistics of different investigations.

Hepatocyte damage with necrotic changes mostly starts with midzonal area and then spreads to centrilobular area. As these particular areas are more sensitive to anoxic or immune-mediated injury [7, 8].

5. Clinical presentation with liver involvement in dengue fever

Clinical evidence suggests that dengue-related hepatic involvement incudes the presence of liver enlargement. Among the clinical features of hepatic involvement, patients have abdominal pain (18–63%) and nausea/vomiting (49–58%). Abdominal pain and anorexia are more common in DF than DHF [12].

Hepatomegaly can be seen in both DF and DHF but more common in DF. The incidence of hepatomegaly in the adult patients varies from 4 to 52%. Clinical jaundice has been found in only 1.7–17%, and hyperbilirubinemia has been found to be as high as 48% [13, 14].

5.1. Biochemical picture of liver (LFTs) in dengue fever

The most common abnormality has been raised transaminases levels. The raised aspartate transaminase (AST) levels are found around 63–97% of patients, whereas the elevated alanine transaminase (ALT) levels are found in 45–96% of patients [8].

Studies have shown in majority of cases that aspartate transaminase (AST) is usually more raised than alanine transaminase (ALT), more during the early infection, especially within first week and then declining to normal levels in next 3 weeks. Aspartate transaminase (AST) is more raised than alanine transaminase (ALT), the additional aspartate transaminase (AST) is released from damaged myocyte.

The reversal of alanine transaminase and aspartate transaminase (AST/ALT) ratio is helpful to differentiate it from other acute viral hepatitis like HAV, HBV, HCV, etc., where this is rarely seen except in alcoholic hepatitis [6].

The average levels of aspartate transaminase (AST) ranged from 93.3 to 174 U/L while alanine transaminase (ALT) from 86 to 88.5 U/L. The level of increase in hepatic transaminases can easily mimic acute viral hepatitis.

5.2. Role of transaminases as marker of severity of dengue fever

The median aspartate transaminase (AST) and alanine transaminase (ALT) values have been found to be higher for severer forms of dengue than for uncomplicated dengue fever [15].

This hints at a possible association between increased transaminase levels with increasing disease severity. Interestingly, the values of liver enzymes were noted to be higher in the febrile and the severer phases of dengue fever.

Aspartate transaminase (AST) has various sources including the heart, striated muscle, erythrocytes, etc., apart from the liver, whilst alanine transaminase (ALT) primarily is hepatic in origin. Therefore, rise in aspartate transaminase (AST) might not be a true reflection of hepatic involvement. Moreover, patients with high levels of enzymes may be labeled as severe disease without any effect on the final outcomes [16].

Hypoproteinemia or hypoalbuminemia ranges from 16.5 to 76%. The heterogeneity in the population and severity of the disease may be responsible for such a wide range.

Coagulation abnormalities have been found in multiple studies. International normalized ratio (INR) > 1.5 have been found in 11% of patients, while abnormal prothrombin time (PT), partial thromboplastin time noted in 34–42.5% of the cases [17].

Increasing bleeding episodes have been seen with increasing alanine transaminase and aspartate transaminase (AST/ALT) levels, but correlation between PT and transaminase levels is not found to be strong during the recovery period, which means liver synthetic function like clotting factor production is usually well preserved.

Liver involvement comes commonly and with more severity in children as compared to adults [18]. Treatment is primarily supportive, and the prognosis is usually good. Differential diagnosis and hepatotoxic drugs should be avoided [19].

5.3. Suggestions

Liver function tests should be used as routine initial part of the investigative studies in a patient with suspected dengue fever.

Serial monitoring of liver function tests, especially alanine transaminase (ALT), should be done to identify high-risk cases.

Author details

Ambreen Zubair[1]*, Asim Ahmad Qureshi[2] and Syed Ahmed Murtaza Jafri[3]

*Address all correspondence to: ambreenzubair@gmail.com

1 King Edward Medical University, Lahore, Pakistan

2 WMD, Birmingham, United Kingdom

3 Doctors Institute of Medical Sciences Lahore, Lahore, Pakistan

References

[1] Guzman MG, Halstead SB, Artsob H, Buchy P, Farrar J, Gubler DJ, Hunsperger E, Kroeger A, Margolis HS, Martínez E, et al. Dengue: A continuing global threat. Nature Reviews Microbiology. 2010;**8**:S7–S16.[PMC free article] [PubMed]

[2] Guzmán MG, Kourí G. Dengue: An update. Lancet Infectious Diseases. 2002;**2**:33-42. [PubMed]

[3] Thomas SJ, Strickman D, Vaughn DW. Dengue epidemiology: Virus epidemiology, ecology, and emergence. Advances in Virus Research. 2003;**61**:235-289. [PubMed]

[4] WHO. Dengue Hemorrhagic Fever: Diagnosis, Treatment, Prevention and Control, Geneva [Internet]. 1997. Available from: http://www.who.int/csr/resources/publications/dengue/Denguepublication/en/

[5] Chang K, Lu PL, Ko WC, et al. Dengue fever scoring system: New strategy for the early detection of acute dengue virus infection in Taiwan. Journal of the Formosan Medical Association. 2009;**108**:879-885

[6] Lee LK, Gan VC, Lee VJ, Tan AS, Leo YS, Lye DC. Clinical relevance and discriminatory value of elevated liver aminotransferase levels for dengue severity. PLoS Neglected Tropical Diseases. 2012;**6**:e1676.[PMC free article] [PubMed]

[7] Seneviratne SL, Malavige GN, de Silva HJ. Pathogenesis of liver involvement during dengue viral infections. Transactions of the Royal Society of Tropical Medicine and Hygiene. 2006;**100**:608-614. [PubMed]

[8] Huerre MR, Lan NT, Marianneau P, Hue NB, Khun H, Hung NT, Khen NT, Drouet MT, Huong VT, Ha DQ, et al. Liver histopathology and biological correlates in five cases of fatal dengue fever in Vietnamese children. Virchows Archiv. 2001;**438**:107-115. [PubMed]

[9] Miller JL, de Wet BJ, Martinez-Pomares L, Radcliffe CM, Dwek RA, Rudd PM, Gordon S. The mannose receptor mediates dengue virus infection of macrophages. PLOS Pathogens. 2008;**4**:e17.[PMC free article] [PubMed]

[10] Martina BE, Koraka P, Osterhaus AD. Dengue virus pathogenesis: An integrated view. Clinical Microbiology Reviews. 2009;**22**:564-581. [PMC free article] [PubMed]

[11] Marianneau P, Steffan AM, Royer C, Drouet MT, Jaeck D, Kirn A, Deubel V. Infection of primary cultures of human Kupffer cells by dengue virus: No viral progeny synthesis, but cytokine production is evident. Journal of Virology. 1999;**73**:5201-5206. [PMC free article] [PubMed]

[12] Couvelard A, Marianneau P, Bedel C, Drouet MT, Vachon F, Hénin D, Deubel V. Report of a fatal case of dengue infection with hepatitis: Demonstration of dengue antigens in hepatocytes and liver apoptosis. Human Pathology. 1999;**30**:1106-1110. [PubMed]

[13] Tan SS, Bujang MA. The clinical features and outcomes of acute liver failure associated with dengue infection in adults: A case series. Brazilian Journal of Infectious Diseases. 2013;**17**:164-169. [PubMed]

[14] Giri S, Sharma V, Agarwal MP, Sharma A. Low mortality during 2008 outbreak of dengue in Delhi, India: A clinicobiochemical study. Revista de Ciências Médicas e Biológicas. 2010;**9**:10-12

[15] Kuo CH, Tai DI, Chang-Chien CS, Lan CK, Chiou SS, Liaw YF. Liver biochemical tests and dengue fever. American Journal of Tropical Medicine and Hygiene. 1992;**47**:265-270. [PubMed]

[16] Wong M, Shen E. The utility of liver function tests in dengue. Annals of the Academy of Medicine, Singapore. 2008;**37**:82-83. [PubMed]

[17] Wahid SF, Sanusi S, Zawawi MM, Ali RA. A comparison of the pattern of liver involvement in dengue hemorrhagic fever with classic dengue fever. Southeast Asian Journal of Tropical Medicine and Public Health. 2000;**31**:259-263.[PubMed]

[18] Kulkarni MJ, Sarathi V, Bhalla V, Shivpuri D, Acharya U. Clinico-epidemiological profile of children hospitalized with dengue. The Indian Journal of Pediatrics. 2010;77:1103-1107. [PubMed]

[19] Roy A, Sarkar D, Chakraborty S, Chaudhuri J, Ghosh P, Chakraborty S. Profile of hepatic involvement by dengue virus in dengue infected children. North American Journal of Medical Sciences. 2013;**5**:480-485. [PMC free article][PubMed]

Section 2

Diagnosis

Chapter 4

Diagnosis of Dengue: Strengths and Limitations of Current Techniques and Prospects for Future Improvements

Narayan Gyawali and Andrew W. Taylor-Robinson

Additional information is available at the end of the chapter

http://dx.doi.org/10.5772/67680

Abstract

Dengue is an increasingly common mosquito-borne, flaviviral disease of significant public health concern. The disease is endemic throughout tropical and subtropical regions, placing almost half of the world's population at risk, and each year approaching 100 million people in around 130 countries are infected. There is acknowledged to be four antigenically distinct serotypes of the virus, and arguably a fifth, each of which elicits a full spectrum of clinical disease. This ranges from asymptomatic self-limiting infection to life-threatening severe manifestations characterized by plasma leakage, bleeding, and/or organ failure. Recovery from primary infection by one serotype provides lifelong immunity against reinfection by that particular serotype, whereas with subsequent infections by other serotypes, the risk of developing severe dengue is increased. Rising mortality and morbidity rates caused by infection in recent years are attributable partly to a lack of availability of effective antiviral therapies and vaccines. In this context, early detection of infection with sensitive and specific laboratory tools and the prompt clinical management of this disease is a health care priority. Although a variety of techniques are currently used for laboratory diagnosis of dengue, no single methodology satisfies the ideal requirement for both sensitivity and specificity, while also being rapid and inexpensive. Newer detection tools that can fill this acknowledged gap in dengue diagnosis are urgently required.

Keywords: dengue, virus, diagnosis, serotype, antibody, nucleic acid, PCR

1. Introduction

Dengue is a mosquito-borne viral disease that has a wide-ranging geographical distribution throughout the tropics and subtropics. It is estimated that currently over 3.9 billion people are at risk of infection [1], with 96 million notified clinical cases per year in at least 128 countries worldwide [2]. Dengue virus (DENV) is transmitted by mosquitoes of the *Aedes* genus, primarily *Ae. aegypti,* but also *Ae. albopictus* and *Ae. polynesiensis* [3]. DENV is a member of the family *Flaviviridae* [4], which also includes the other major human pathogens West Nile, yellow fever, Zika, Japanese encephalitis, and tick-borne encephalitis viruses. Four serotypes of the virus (DENV-1 to DENV-4) have been known for many years, while a putative fifth serotype, DENV-5, was identified recently [5]. This new subtype was identified during screening tests on virus samples collected during an outbreak in Malaysia in 2007 [6].

DENV infection may result in a progressive scope of clinical sequelae, viewed traditionally as ranging from asymptomatic infection through to dengue fever (DF) and the more severe disease manifestations of dengue haemorrhagic fever (DHF) and dengue shock syndrome (DSS). More recently [7], the World Health Organization proposed a revised classification that categorizes infection as follows: (1) dengue; (2) dengue with warning signs (abdominal pain, persistent vomiting, fluid accumulation, mucosal bleeding, lethargy, liver enlargement, and increasing hematocrit with decreasing platelets); and (3) severe dengue (dengue with severe plasma leakage, severe bleeding, and/or organ failure). Asymptomatic infections are characterized by undifferentiated fever with or without rashes. In the majority of clinical cases, the initial presentation of dengue is not apparent until clear signs and symptoms develop. In turn, this delay limits the ability to make an early and accurate clinical diagnosis. Moreover, there are no specific therapies for dengue, such as anti-viral drugs. Any treatment is essentially supportive, and thus, there is a very important challenge in making an informed estimate of the severity of a patient's disease as early as is practicable. The preliminary stages of DF are often confused with other febrile tropical diseases [8], which may lead to inappropriate therapy.

Although very recently, the first licensed dengue vaccine (DENV-1 to DENV-4 chimera constructed on a yellow fever 17D backbone, recombinant, live attenuated, tetravalent virus (CYD-TDV; Dengvaxia®, Sanofi Pasteur)) has been registered for use [9], major challenges to vaccine effectiveness and long-term safety in the administered population remain. This scenario, therefore, still demands a quick and reliable diagnostic approach. While a variety of laboratory diagnostic techniques have been in use for many years, each has its limitations [10], to date no tool proving to be reliable, rapid, and cost-effective. There is, therefore, a pressing need to improve the way in which dengue is diagnosed. The overall scenario calls for the development of reliable and rapid dengue diagnostic tools.

2. Current laboratory methods for dengue diagnosis

2.1. Virus isolation

Virus isolation is considered to be the gold standard technique in dengue diagnosis [11]. Isolation is highly successful when specimens are collected in the viraemic period, which starts 2–3 days before the onset of fever and lasts for a further 2–3 days [12]. Routinely, serum is the primary choice of sample. In addition, other types of specimen, including plasma, peripheral blood, cerebrospinal fluid, pleural fluid, and tissues of reticuloendothelial origin such as liver, spleen, lymph nodes, lung, and thymus, are of substantial importance [7, 12, 13]. Diagnostic sensitivity is dependent upon the timing of specimen collection, proper storage, and transportation. Since the DENV virus particle is heat-labile, appropriate handling and prompt delivery to the laboratory is required. When storage is warranted, a standard refrigerator temperature (~4°C) is quite appropriate in the short term, while for a longer duration, freezer temperatures of −20 or −70°C are recommended. In the latter case, they should be maintained in order to prevent thawing [13].

There are different methods available for the isolation of DENV including inoculation of specimens into mosquitoes (adults or larvae); various *in vitro* insect or mammalian cell cultures; and injection intra-cerebrally in mice [12, 14–16].

2.1.1. *Specimen inoculation into mosquitoes*

Inoculation of specimens into both adult and larval mosquitoes with the objective to isolate DENV is considered to be the most sensitive and specific culture technique. Generally, mosquitoes belonging to the *Toxorhynchites* genus are used for this purpose. The advantage of these over *Aedes* mosquitoes is that the former has an unusual life cycle in not being hematophagous, so may be handled with impunity. In addition, the comparatively larger size of *Toxorhynchites* facilitates easier introduction of inocula. However, the fact that between 5 and 20 mosquitoes are needed to produce results of higher sensitivity is considered a drawback of this method. Alternatively, adult male *Ae. aegypti* and *Ae. albopictus* mosquitoes are also useful for virus isolation [17, 18]. The preferred route for specimen inoculation of mosquitoes is intrathoracic. Incubation for 14 days at 32°C following inoculation precedes mosquito storage at −70°C [19]. Successful virus infection of mosquitoes is confirmed by the detection of antigen in a smear prepared by crushing of mosquito heads on a microscope slide followed by serotype-specific immunofluorescence. A preparation of thorax-abdomens can also be tested for virus by plaque assay or plaque reduction neutralization test (PRNT) using monospecific dengue virus antisera targeted against different DENV serotypes [20]. The labor-intensive process of raising mosquitoes requires arranging for a second mosquito species to serve as a food source (because *Toxorhynchites* mosquitoes are carnivorous). In addition, the requirement for facilities with capacity to rear and handle infectious *Aedes* mosquitoes while adhering to stringent health and safety protocols is beyond the capability of most laboratories and remains a major obstacle. Similarly, the need for both specialist containment and highly skilled technicians in order to perform direct mosquito inoculation has combined to make *in vitro* cell culture a preferred option [21].

2.1.2. *Mosquito or mammalian cell line culture*

In vitro culture of cell lines is a technique being developed as an alternative tool for virus isolation and aimed at overcoming the pitfalls involved in mosquito inoculation. However, thus far the variety of approaches to cell line culture is limited by the lower sensitivity of results obtained. Cell line cultures from *Ae. albopictus* (C6/36), *Ae. pseudoscutelaris* (AP-61,

AP-64), and *Tinissa amboinensis* (TRA-284) are different choices for routine DENV isolation [22–24]. All three of these have distinct benefits and drawbacks, so preference of use should be made on a case-by-case basis. In a comparative study, the virus isolation rate was found to be highest in TRA-284, followed by AP-61 and C6/36 [24]. In contrast, C6/36 cells were preferable for detecting infected cells by the direct fluorescent antibody test (DFAT). The utility of the C6/36 cell line method to isolate virus from tissue samples derived from fatal cases of dengue has been demonstrated [16]. Problems with AP-61 and TRA-284 include frequent cell clumping and difficulties in formation of a monolayer in a tissue culture flask. Some dengue viruses, especially wild types, do not produce cytopathic effects on these cell lines [24], which limits usage of the plaque assay and PRNT for virus quantification and virus-neutralizing antibody detection. Therefore, for specific diagnosis, immunoassays should be used.

Alternatives for isolating virus are mammalian cells such as Vero and BS-C-1 (both derived from African green monkey kidney), LLCMK2 rhesus monkey kidney, PS (porcine kidney), and BHK 21 (baby hamster kidney). While these cell cultures are used widely in the PRNT, they produce less sensitive results. PRNT is considered as the benchmark means to characterize and quantify circulating levels of anti-DENV neutralizing antibody [25–27].

2.1.3. Intra-cerebral injection in mice

The oldest and least sensitive method for virus isolation is intracerebral inoculation of suckling mice. This does, nonetheless, offer a considerable benefit in enabling evaluation of the neutrotropic characteristics of the dengue virus particle *in vivo*. In most cases, mice develop encephalitis symptoms [28]. However, virus identification is generally accomplished by immunofluorescence methods with serotype-specific anti-dengue antibodies applied to infected cells or brain tissue of mice. This is a cumbersome procedure, and the need for a high specification laboratory microscope combined with difficulties in maintaining viability of the virus in specimens limit its use on a routine basis.

2.2. Viral nucleic acid detection

DENV is a single-stranded positive-sense RNA virus of approximately 50 nm in length. The 11 kb genome of each virion encodes three structural proteins (capsid, C; precursor membrane, prM; and envelope, E) and seven non-structural (NS) proteins (NS1, NS2A, NS2B, NS3, NS4A, NS4B, and NS5). These non-structural proteins play roles in viral replication and assembly. Structurally, a virion consists of a nucleocapsid, enveloped by an outer glycoprotein shell and an inner lipid bilayer. Surface projections in the lipid membrane consist of E and membrane (M) glycoproteins [4].

Nucleic acid amplification tests and identification of virus antigen or antibody serve as the predominant means of detection of DENV, based on the molecular or immunological response to specified viral structural components. Commonly used methods are reverse transcription polymerase chain reaction (RT-PCR), nucleic acid sequence-based amplification (NASBA), and transcription-mediated amplification (TMA).

2.2.1. Polymerase chain reaction

Virus RNA genome detection tests are faster and considered more sensitive than virus isolation and its detection. Thoughtful design of primer sequence may be applied to not only distinguish the binary presence of the target virus but also determine detailed features of the viral genome such as serotype or polymorphisms. Type-specific primers and consensus sequences that are located in different genes of most flaviviruses including dengue, such as those for E, NS1, NS3, and NS5, have been used extensively for the detection and identification of DENV [29–32]. For a PCR run, DENV RNA should pass through a conversion step to complementary DNA (cDNA) by a process of reverse transcription (RT). Conventional PCR can be used to identify the presence or absence of a target sequence in a given sample when reaction products are visualized by agarose gel electrophoresis [33], Southern blot [34], or colorimetric enzyme-linked immunosorbent assay [35]. While easy to enact, these conventional procedures have a limited inference in comparison to more versatile PCR systems. They are considered less robust as multiple handling steps are required, which increase the risk of contamination and hence the production of false-positive results.

Modification of protocols to make use of nested primers aims to reduce non-specific detection by negating improper primer binding. In nested PCR, targets are detected by using two sets of primers involving a double process of amplification. However, the greater manipulation of the sample that this technique involves may raise the risk of contamination of the amplicon product. Multiplex PCR is an adaptation that allows simultaneous amplification and detection of multiple target amplicons, which can be used to great effect in distinguishing conditions such as viral serotype. Both methods have been found to increase the sensitivity and specificity of the test and are preferred for the diagnosis of DENV [33, 36].

Real-time PCR, also known as quantitative PCR (qPCR), is a far more robust assay format than conventional PCR, over which it has many advantages including rapidity, quantitative measurements, lower contamination rate, higher sensitivity, and specificity, and ease of standardization. Furthermore, qPCR renders post-PCR procedures such as electrophoresis or blotting unnecessary, minimizing the chance of contamination. As per conventional PCR, qPCR primer sequence can be specified to detect specific DENV to a threshold that is usually less than 100 plaque-forming units [33, 37].

With advances in diagnosis, the two-step nested RT-PCR protocol, modified to a single-step multiplex RT-PCR for detection and typing of DENV, is well established [33]. In nested PCR, targets are detected by using two sets of primers involving a double process of amplification. A nested PCR assay was developed using DENV consensus primers located in the C and prM genes that amplify a 511-bp product in a reverse transcriptase PCR followed by a nested PCR with primers specific to each DENV serotype [33]. Application of multiplex qPCR for the diagnosis of dengue has been described by various studies [36–38]. Each has concluded that this technique demonstrates superior analytical and clinical performance, as well as simpler workflow, than the heminested RT-PCR [38]. More recently, several investigators have reported on fully automatic real-time RT-PCR assays for the detection of DENV in acute-phase serum samples [39–43].

2.2.2. Nucleic acid sequence-based amplification

Nucleic acid sequence-based amplification (NASBA) is a one-step transcription-mediated isothermal process for amplifying RNA. Throughout the amplification reaction, a constant temperature of 41°C is maintained. The reaction mixture contains three enzymes: avian myeloblastosis reverse transcriptase (AMV-RT); T7 RNA polymerase; and RNase H with two short, single-stranded DNA primers. Multiple transcription of RNA copies of DNA products that are produced from the initial reverse transcription step are attributable for the exponential kinetics of NASBA. Hence, synthesized RNA pools are detected by fluorescence. These "molecular beacons" are single-stranded hairpin-shaped oligonucleotide probes showing fluorescence at the 5′ end and with a fluorescence quencher at the 3′ end. When presented in an amplification reaction with their amplified target RNA, a stable hybrid is formed [44].

Studies have found a sensitivity of 98.5% and specificity of 100% when they detected DENV with NASBA [45, 46]. The effectiveness of this method has also been described for detecting dengue virus within mosquitoes [47]. It is considered more efficient than PCR in that it bypasses the use of a thermal cycler, which makes it both cost-effective and rapid (<1 day).

2.2.3. Reverse transcription loop-mediated isothermal amplification

Loop-mediated isothermal amplification (LAMP) is a novel PCR method that is based on the principle of a strand displacement reaction involving a stem loop structure that amplifies the target genome [48]. Its advantage over other amplification methods is the ease of monitoring of amplification; pyrophosphate ions produced as a by-product of reaction substrate deoxynucleotide triphosphates form a white precipitate of magnesium pyrophosphate that can be visualized by the naked eye, measured by turbidometer, detected by hand-held UV torch, or even following staining with SYBR green® or ethidium bromide [49, 50]. Furthermore, it takes less than one hour to yield results compared to the 3–4 h typically needed to run RT-PCR [51].

Several studies have found RT-LAMP to be a superior tool to RT-PCR in terms of sensitivity and specificity for detection and accurate differentiation of flaviviruses [49, 50, 52, 53]. Sensitivity of the tool is variously reported at 100% [49, 52, 54], with a lowest detection limit of 100 copy numbers of RNAs, while specificity ranges from 87.5 to 100% [49, 50, 52, 53].

2.3. Serological methods

2.3.1. Antigen detection

During the febrile phase of dengue illness, DENV antigens may be detected in peripheral blood leukocytes, liver [54], and lung at autopsy, and less often in the thymus, lymph nodes, skin, spleen [55], bone marrow, and serosa [56]. Immunohistochemistry and enzyme immunoassay (EIA) are useful techniques to detect dengue antigens in tissue sections (frozen, paraffin-embedded) using labeled monoclonal antibodies that are visualized with markers such as fluorescent dyes (fluorescent antibody), enzymes (immunoperoxidase and avidin-biotin enzyme) or colloidal gold. Given the inconvenience of collecting samples on which to apply these techniques, their utility has been limited for routine laboratory tests. Instead, assays have been developed against intact virus particle and recombinant viral proteins, with NS1 and E protein detection available commercially [57, 58].

2.3.2. Non-structural proteins (NS1 and NS5)-based assay

Non-structural gene, NS1, is a highly conserved glycoprotein produced by all flaviviruses in both membrane-associated and secreted forms, and which is essential for viral replication and viability [59]. Localized to cellular organelles, this antigen is secreted abundantly in sera of patients during virus replication and the early stage of infection [58]. A unique feature of this protein is its secretion by mammalian cells as hexamers (dimer subunits only), while it is not secreted by insect cells, including those of mosquitoes. Glycosylation is believed to be an important step for protein secretion. It can be identified in peripheral blood prior to formation of antibodies, and the detection rate is higher in acute primary infection from the day of onset of fever to day 9 [60, 61]. NS1 is also a complement-fixing antigen that elicits a very strong humoral response.

Several recent studies have addressed the use of NS1 antigen and anti-NS1 antibodies as a tool for dengue diagnosis [62–65], with higher specificity for determination of homologous serotypes by serotype- and group-specific NS1 capture ELISA [62, 66], and a detection sensitivity of 1–4 ng/ml NS1 in blood [67]. This tool can be utilized to differentiate between primary and secondary dengue virus infections, as proven by the highly correlated results of NS1 serotype-specific IgG (determined by ELISA) and PRNT [43, 68]. The NS1 serotype-specific IgG ELISA worked reliably for serotyping dengue virus in convalescent phase sera from patients with primary infection and also in acute phase sera from patients with secondary infection (in which the serotype that caused the first infection would be detected), but not so with convalescent phase sera from patients with secondary infections. Different commercial assays to detect NS1 antigen are available, including Panbio dengue virus Pan-E NS1 early ELISA (Alere); dengue virus NS1 antigen ELISA (Standard Diagnostics); Platelia NS1 antigen ELISA (Bio-Rad). However, none of these have excellent sensitivity, ranging from 45 to 57% [69]. NS1 ELISA has a noted lower sensitivity in sera from patients infected with DENV-4. This may be due to possible quantitative differences in the secretion of NS1 antigen by distinct serotypes [70].

Dengue non-structural protein NS5, which plays a vital role in dengue replication, is the largest and most well conserved of the flavivirus proteins [71]. One study demonstrated reliable results in diagnosing and differentiating DENV from West Nile virus and St. Louis encephalitis (SLE) virus using an immunoassay designed to targeting NS5 antigen [72]. However, questions arise as to its specificity since NS5 amino acid sequence homology between West Nile, dengue, and SLE viruses is more than 75% [72], hence a greater chance that results would be affected by cross-reactivity.

2.4. Antibody detection

DENV-specific IgM antibodies start to appear after 4–5 days of primary infection and are measurable for up to 3 months [73]. IgG antibodies appear about a week after onset of fever, persist at high titres for several weeks and then decline; however, IgG may be detected for decades [74]. IgG1 and IgG3 are the subclasses that are mainly induced [75, 76]. Following secondary infection, memory B cells are stimulated in response to secrete DENV-specific IgG that is measurable even on the first day of symptoms and the titre remains much higher compared to during primary infection. In secondary dengue, the IgM response is variable and, in some cases, even undetectable. The most commonly used antibody detection techniques for dengue diagnosis are haemagglutination inhibition (HI) and ELISA for IgM or IgG [77].

2.4.1. Hemagglutination inhibition

The hemagglutination inhibition (HI) method was a routinely utilized method before the development of the fast and easier antibody detection methods immunofluorescence assay (IFA) and ELISA. Due to its high degree of sensitivity and ease of application, HI is still used sometimes in developing countries. The test is based on the principle whereby the property of erythrocyte agglutination by dengue proteins is inhibited when dengue antibodies are present in serum at a sufficient concentration [78]. The most important practical limitations of the HI test are its poor specificity, requirement for paired samples, and the inability to distinguish dengue serotype [35]. Moreover, the test fails to differentiate dengue from the closely related Japanese encephalitis and yellow fever flaviviruses [11, 78, 79].

2.4.2. E/M-specific capture IgM and IgG ELISA

Methods of detection of dengue by capturing E/M-specific IgM and IgG antibodies are relatively efficient in terms of their higher diagnostic sensitivity, specificity, simplicity, and feasibility of use in low-resource countries where facilities for molecular diagnosis are not standardly available [80–82].

In IgM antibody capture (MAC)-ELISA, the total IgM in a patient's sera is bound by anti-μ chain-specific antibodies precoated on the microtitre plate [83]. Due to its rapid production then gradual waning after 2–3 months ELISA based on IgM detection is considered sensitive in early dengue infection, while not being suitable in cases of prolonged infection [11, 84].

E/M-specific IgG antibody capture ELISA, also called GAC-ELISA, enables measurement of IgG for up to 10 months after infection, thereby facilitating detection of recent and past dengue infection. In general, IgG ELISA lacks specificity within the flavivirus sero-complex groups; however, the IgG response to prM is specific to individual flaviviruses [85]. Dengue secondary infection progresses to severe dengue, so it is important to differentiate secondary from primary infection. IgG avidity ELISAs can be used to determine whether an infection is primary or secondary [86, 87]. The principle behind this method is that antibodies first synthesized after primary infection exhibit a lower affinity for antigen than do those produced later during secondary infection.

Classification of primary and secondary infections can also be defined in terms of the ratio of anti-DENV IgM to IgG antibodies. A higher IgM/IgG ratio specifies the infection as being primary, for which a ratio value of 1.2 is considered as a distinguishing cut-off. However, the most reliable way to demonstrate active infection would be a significant (fourfold or greater) rise in IgM and/or IgG antibody titres between acute and convalescent phase sera [88].

Cross-reactivity between flavivirus antigens is the major issue that lowers the specificity of ELISA. While this may be reduced by detecting E/M- and NS1-specific anti-dengue virus IgM antibodies, E/M-specific IgG elicited by different flavivirus sero-complexes are highly cross-reactive [10, 11]. In order to increase the specificity of results analysis of paired serum samples from both acute and convalescent phases is strongly recommended [10, 11].

2.5. Rapid diagnostic test

Immunochromatographic tests are developed to meet the need for rapid methods of dengue diagnosis. The value of the immunochromatographic format is its rapid attainment of a result by virtue of a color change that is visible to the naked eye within 10–15 min. Tools are based on the detection of anti-dengue IgM and IgG antibodies and of dengue antigens. A number of studies have evaluated dengue rapid diagnostic tests (RDTs) [89–93]. Commonly used RDTs are Duo IgM and IgG Rapid Test Strip (Panbio); Bioline Dengue IgG/IgM (Standard Diagnostics); VScan (Minerava); Smartcheck (GlobaleMed); Denguecheck-WB (Tulip); and Dengue IgG/IgM (Core). With acute phase samples, the diagnostic accuracy of the tests has not been established reliably, but manufacturers' claimed performance ranges from 76 to 100% sensitivity and exceeding 99% specificity. In contrast, markedly different results were claimed independently [92], suggesting most RDTs are unsuitable for dengue diagnosis as they have poor sensitivity and specificity. A preliminary trial of dengue from Nepal has reported a similar finding when rapid immunochromatographic tests are comparing with ELISA; the former tool did not prove sufficiently reliable with regard to either sensitivity or specificity [82]. In order to overcome the limitations posed by RDTs, techniques have been modified whereby dengue NS1 antigen is detected in combination with anti-glycoprotein E IgM and IgG antibodies [94].

2.6. Dengue virus serotyping and genotyping

Detection and serotyping of dengue viruses are performed by molecular methods such as PCR (nested, semi-nested, and multiplex RT-PCR) using serotype-specific primers [95, 96]. Following RT-PCR, the amplified product is subjected to nucleotide sequencing. The most commonly used commercial sequencing technique for amplicon purification and sequencing is QIAquick PCR Purification Kit (Qiagen). Both strands of the PCR product are sequenced in order to avoid discrepancies. Gene sequences obtained for DENV strains are submitted to the GenBank database (http://www.ncbi.nlm.nih.gov). A basic local alignment search tool (BLAST) algorithm performed against information stored in the database finds regions of local similarity between nucleotide sequences. This may yield functional and evolutionary clues about the structure and function of any novel sequence.

3. Diagnostic limitations

A lack of sensitive, specific, rapid, and cost-effective assays remains the major hurdle to the development of diagnostic tools for dengue virus detection. Although virus isolation is more specific, it is limited by being time-consuming and expensive, needing expertise, an inability to differentiate primary and secondary infections, and requiring acute samples (0–5 days post onset of fever) [13]. Nucleic acid (RNA) detection, although sufficiently sensitive and specific to identify both serotype and genotype in a short time is also restricted by the need for an acute sample, skilled handling, and by its incapacity to distinguish primary from secondary infections [78]. Furthermore, it is an expensive tool that is not affordable by all laboratories. While these limitations are being overcome by the detection of NS1 antigen, its sensitivity compared to genome detection methods is poor and cannot be guaranteed [68]. Tests that measure anti-dengue IgM antibodies are useful only for the first 4–6 days of infection. Also, IgM levels in secondary infection are quite low and could be below the threshold for detection. Moreover, IgG specificity is reduced due to cross-reactivity among flaviviruses [10, 11, 97].

4. Future directions

Challenges in developing a highly sensitive and specific diagnostic tool should be addressed. Possibilities for improvement lie in combining current techniques that could enhance both sensitivity and specificity. A rapid, sensitive test that combines detection of NS1, IgG, and IgM, thereby enabling diagnosis of infection throughout the course of illness, would provide a significant advancement in dengue diagnostics.

A potential tool to detect dengue is based on detection of the light transmission spectrum recorded in the near-infrared range (NIR). NIR spectroscopy is a fast, multicomponent assay that enables non-invasive, non-destructive analysis, in this case of human blood samples. NIR spectroscopy has become a widely used analytical method in the agricultural, chemical, petrochemical, pharmaceutical, and medical industries [98]. It may also find an application in the medical diagnostics field and preliminary investigations are underway. In general, optical spectroscopy is a technique that utilizes the light energy-dependent interaction with a sample (electromagnetic radiation usually quantified by wavelength). Biological substances can interact with light energy and produce a variety of optical responses—transmission, reflection scattering, and absorption. By scanning C6/36 cells either infected or not infected with DENV and/or mouse monoclonal hybridoma antibodies against DENV, differences in NIR spectra may indicate dengue infection. Analysis and standardization of these optical responses could literally help to shed light on dengue diagnosis in the future.

Considerable research has been performed to develop biosensors as effective tools for infectious disease diagnostics [99, 100]. A biosensor based on silicon nanowire can detect the 'reverse transcription polymerase chain reaction' product of dengue in less than 30 min. Peptide nucleic acid probes fixed in silicon nanowires recognize complementary DNA fragments [100]. Sensitive and specific results from these techniques could offset the other labor-intensive and time-consuming laboratory tests requiring trained laboratory staff.

http://dx.doi.org/10.5772/67680

Acknowledgements

The authors' research is supported by Central Queensland University and the Australian Government's Collaborative Research Networks Program.

Author details

Narayan Gyawali[1,2] and Andrew W. Taylor-Robinson[2]*

*Address all correspondence to: a.taylor-robinson@cqu.edu.au

1 WHO Collaborating Centre for Arbovirus Reference and Research, Institute of Health and Biomedical Innovation, Queensland University of Technology, Brisbane, Australia

2 Infectious Diseases Research Group, School of Health, Medical & Applied Sciences, Central Queensland University, Brisbane, Australia

References

[1] Brady OJ, Gething PW, Bhatt S, Messina JP, Brownstein JS, Hoen AG, Moyes CL, Farlow AW, Scott TW, Hay SI. Refining the global spatial limits of dengue virus transmission by evidence-based consensus. PLoS Neglected Tropical Diseases. 2012; **6**: e1760.

[2] Bhatt S, Gething PW, Brady OJ, Messina JP, Farlow AW, Moyes CL, Drake JM, Brownstein JS, Hoen AG, Sankoh O, Myers MF, George DB, Jaenisch T, Wint GR, Simmons CP, Scott TW, Farrar JJ, Hay SI. The global distribution and burden of dengue. Nature. 2013; **496**: 504-507.

[3] Higa Y. Dengue vectors and their spatial distribution. Tropical Medicine and Health. 2011; **39 (suppl. 4)**: 17-27.

[4] Henchal EA, Putnak JR. The dengue viruses. Clinical Microbiology Reviews. 1990; **3**: 376-396.

[5] Normile D. Surprising new dengue virus throws a spanner in disease control efforts. Science. 2013; **342**: 415.

[6] Taylor-Robinson AW. A putative fifth serotype of dengue—potential implications for diagnosis, therapy and vaccine design. International Journal of Clinical & Medical Microbiology. 2016; **1**: 101-102.

[7] World Health Organization. Dengue: Guidelines for Diagnosis, Treatment, Prevention and Control. Geneva: WHO; 2009. 147 p.

[8] George R, Lum LC. Clinical spectrum of dengue infection. In: Gubler DJ, Kuno G, editors. Dengue and Dengue Hemorrhagic Fever. Oxford: CAB International; 1997. pp. 89-114.

[9] Pitisuttithum P, Bouckenooghe A. The first licensed dengue vaccine: an important tool for integrated preventive strategies against dengue virus infection. Expert Review of Vaccines. 2016; **15**: 795-798.

[10] Peeling RW, Artsob H, Pelegrino JL, Buchy P, Cardosa MJ, Devi S, Enria DA, Farrar J, Gubler DJ, Guzman MG, Halstead SB, Hunsperger E, Kliks S, Margolis HS, Nathanson CM, Nguyen VC, Rizzo N, Vázquez S, Yoksan S. Evaluation of diagnostic tests: dengue. Nature Reviews Microbiology. 2010; **8 (suppl. 12)**: S30–S37.

[11] Shu P-Y, Huang J-H. Current advances in dengue diagnosis. Clinical and Diagnostic Laboratory Immunology. 2004; **11**: 642-650.

[12] Vorndam V, Kuno G, Gubler D, Kuno G. Laboratory diagnosis of dengue virus infections. In: Gubler DJ, Kuno G, editors. Dengue and Dengue Hemorrhagic Fever. Oxford: CAB International; 1997. pp. 313-333.

[13] Guzmán MG, Kourí G. Dengue diagnosis, advances and challenges. International Journal of Infectious Diseases. 2004; **8**: 69-80.

[14] Kimura R. Studies on dengue fever (VI). On the inoculation of dengue virus into mice. Nippon Igaku. 1944; **3379**: 629-633.

[15] Rosen L. The use of *Toxorhynchites* mosquitoes to detect and propagate dengue and other arboviruses. American Journal of Tropical Medicine and Hygiene. 1981; **30**: 177-183.

[16] Lam S-K, Chew C-B, Poon G-K, Ramalingam S, Seow S-C, Pang T. Isolation of dengue viruses by intracerebral inoculation of mosquito larvae. Journal of Virological Methods. 1986; **14**: 133-140.

[17] Rosen L, Gubler D. The use of mosquitoes to detect and propagate dengue viruses. American Journal of Tropical Medicine and Hygiene. 1974; **23**: 1153-1160.

[18] Collins LE, Blackwell A. The biology of *Toxorhynchites* mosquitoes and their potential as biocontrol agents. Biocontrol News and Information. 2000; **21**: 105N–116N.

[19] Choy MM, Ellis BR, Ellis EM, Gubler DJ. Comparison of the mosquito inoculation technique and quantitative real time polymerase chain reaction to measure dengue virus concentration. American Journal of Tropical Medicine and Hygiene. 2013; **89**: 1001-1005.

[20] Watts DM, Harrison BA, Nisalak A, Scott RM, Burke DS. Evaluation of *Toxorhynchites splendens* (Diptera: Culicidae) as a bioassay host for dengue viruses. Journal of Medical Entomology. 1982; **19**: 54-59.

[21] Philip Samuel P, Tyagi B. Diagnostic methods for detection & isolation of dengue viruses from vector mosquitoes. Indian Journal of Medical Research. 2006; **123**: 615-628.

[22] Singh KRP, Paul SD. Multiplication of arboviruses in cell lines from *Aedes albopictus* and *Aedes aegypti*. Current Science. 1968; **37**: 65-67.

[23] Race MW, Fortune RA, Agostini C, Varma M. Isolation of dengue viruses in mosquito cell cultures under field conditions. Lancet. 1978; **1**: 48-49.

[24] Kuno G, Gubler D, Vélez M, Oliver A. Comparative sensitivity of three mosquito cell lines for isolation of dengue viruses. Bulletin of the World Health Organization. 1985; **63**: 279-286.

[25] Halstead SB, Sukhavachana P, Nisalak A. Assay of mouse adapted dengue viruses in mammalian cell cultures by an interference method. Proceedings of the Society for Experimental Biology and Medicine. 1964; **115**: 1062-1068.

[26] Russell PK, Nisalak A. Dengue virus identification by the plaque reduction neutralization test. Journal of Immunology. 1967; **99**: 291-296.

[27] Thomas SJ, Nisalak A, Anderson KB, Libraty DH, Kalayanarooj S, Vaughn DW, Putnak R, Gibbons RV, Jarman R, Endy TP. Dengue plaque reduction neutralization test (PRNT) in primary and secondary dengue virus infections: how alterations in assay conditions impact performance. American Journal of Tropical Medicine and Hygiene. 2009; **81**: 825-833.

[28] Amaral DC, Rachid MA, Vilela MC, Campos RD, Ferreira GP, Rodrigues DH, Lacerda-Queiroz N, Miranda AS, Costa VV, Campos MA, Kroon EG, Teixeira MM, Teixeira AL. Intracerebral infection with dengue-3 virus induces meningoencephalitis and behavioral changes that precede lethality in mice. Journal of Neuroinflammation. 2011; **8**: 23.

[29] Deubel V, Laille M, Hugnot J-P, Chungue E, Guesdon J-L, Drouet MT, Bassot S, Chevrier D. Identification of dengue sequences by genomic amplification: rapid diagnosis of dengue virus serotypes in peripheral blood. Journal of Virological Methods. 1990; **30**: 41-54.

[30] Chungue E, Roche C, Lefevre MF, Barbazan P, Chanteau S. Ultra-rapid, simple, sensitive, and economical silica method for extraction of dengue viral RNA from clinical specimens and mosquitoes by reverse transcriptase-polymerase chain reaction. Journal of Medical Virology. 1993; **40**: 142-145.

[31] Fulop L, Barrett AD, Phillpotts R, Martin K, Leslie D, Titball RW. Rapid identification of flaviviruses based on conserved NS5 gene sequences. Journal of Virological Methods. 1993; **44**: 179-188.

[32] Suk-Yin C, Kautner IM, Lam S-K. The influence of antibody levels in dengue diagnosis by polymerase chain reaction. Journal of Virological Methods. 1994; **49**: 315-322.

[33] Lanciotti RS, Calisher CH, Gubler DJ, Chang G-J, Vorndam AV. Rapid detection and typing of dengue viruses from clinical samples by using reverse transcriptase-polymerase chain reaction. Journal of Clinical Microbiology. 1992; **30**: 545-551.

[34] Chang G, Trent DW, Vorndam AV, Vergne E, Kinney RM, Mitchell CJ. An integrated target sequence and signal amplification assay, reverse transcriptase-PCR-enzyme-linked immu-

nosorbent assay, to detect and characterize flaviviruses. Journal of Clinical Microbiology. 1994; **32**: 477-483.

[35] De Paula SO, Fonseca BA. Dengue: a review of the laboratory tests a clinician must know to achieve a correct diagnosis. Brazilian Journal of Infectous Diseases. 2004; **8**: 390-398.

[36] Waggoner JJ, Abeynayake J, Sahoo MK, Gresh L, Tellez Y, Gonzalez K, Ballesteros G, Pierro AM, Gaibani P, Guo FP, Sambri V, Balmaseda A, Karunaratne K, Harris E, Pinsky BA. Single-reaction, multiplex, real-time RT-PCR for the detection, quantitation, and serotyping of dengue viruses. PLoS Neglected Tropical Diseases. 2013; **7**: e2116.

[37] Yong YK, Thayan R, Chong HT, Tan CT, Sekaran SD. Rapid detection and serotyping of dengue virus by multiplex RT-PCR and real-time SYBR green RT-PCR. Singapore Medical Journal. 2007; **48**: 662-668.

[38] Mishra B, Sharma M, Pujhari SK, Appannanavar SB, Ratho RK. Clinical applicability of single-tube multiplex reverse-transcriptase PCR in dengue virus diagnosis and serotyping. Journal of Clinical Laboratory Analysis. 2011; **25**: 76-78.

[39] Houng H-SH, Chung-Ming Chen R, Vaughn DW, Kanesa-thasan N. Development of a fluorogenic RT-PCR system for quantitative identification of dengue virus serotypes 1-4 using conserved and serotype-specific 3′ noncoding sequences. Journal of Virological Methods. 2001; **95**: 19-32.

[40] Drosten C, Göttig S, Schilling S, Asper M, Panning M, Schmitz H, Günther S. Rapid detection and quantification of RNA of Ebola and Marburg viruses, Lassa virus, Crimean-Congo hemorrhagic fever virus, Rift Valley fever virus, dengue virus, and yellow fever virus by real-time reverse transcription-PCR. Journal of Clinical Microbiology. 2002; **40**: 2323-2330.

[41] Wang W-K, Sung T-L, Tsai Y-C, Kao C-L, Chang S-M, King C-C. Detection of dengue virus replication in peripheral blood mononuclear cells from dengue virus type 2-infected patients by a reverse transcription-real-time PCR assay. Journal of Clinical Microbiology. 2002; **40**: 4472-4478.

[42] Warrilow D, Northill JA, Pyke A, Smith GA. Single rapid TaqMan fluorogenic probe based PCR assay that detects all four dengue serotypes. Journal of Medical Virology. 2002; **66**: 524-528.

[43] Shu P-Y, Chang S-F, Kuo Y-C, Yueh Y-Y, Chien L-J, Sue C-L, Lin T-H, Huang J-H. Development of group-and serotype-specific one-step SYBR green I-based real-time reverse transcription-PCR assay for dengue virus. Journal of Clinical Microbiology. 2003; **41**: 2408-2416.

[44] Fakruddin M, Mannan KSB, Chowdhury A, Mazumdar RM, Hossain MN, Islam S, Chowdhury MA. Nucleic acid amplification: alternative methods of polymerase chain reaction. Journal of Pharmacy & Bioallied Sciences. 2013; **5**: 245-252.

[45] Wu S-JL, Lee EM, Putvatana R, Shurtliff RN, Porter KR, Suharyono W, Watts DM, King C-C, Murphy GS, Hayes CG, Romano JW. Detection of dengue viral RNA using a nucleic acid sequence-based amplification assay. Journal of Clinical Microbiology. 2001; **39**: 2794-2798.

[46] Usawattanakul W, Jittmittraphap A, Endy TP, Nisalak A, Tapchaisri P, Looareesuwan S. Rapid detection of dengue viral RNA by nucleic acid sequence-based amplification (NASBA). Dengue Bulletin. 2002; **26**: 125-130.

[47] Jittmittraphap A, Thammapalo S, Ratanasetyuth N, Wongba N, Mammen MP, Jampangern W. Rapid detection of dengue viral RNA in mosquitoes by nucleic acid-sequence based amplification (NASBA). Southeast Asian Journal of Tropical Medicine and Public Health. 2006; **37**: 1117-1124.

[48] Notomi T, Okayama H, Masubuchi H, Yonekawa T, Watanabe K, Amino N, Hase T. Loop-mediated isothermal amplification of DNA. Nucleic Acids Research. 2000; **28**: E63.

[49] Parida M, Horioke K, Ishida H, Dash PK, Saxena P, Jana AM, Islam MA, Inoue S, Hosaka N, Morita K. Rapid detection and differentiation of dengue virus serotypes by a real-time reverse transcription-loop-mediated isothermal amplification assay. Journal of Clinical Microbiology. 2005; **43**: 2895-2903.

[50] Sahni AK, Grover N, Sharma A, Khan ID, Kishore J. Reverse transcription loop-mediated isothermal amplification (RT-LAMP) for diagnosis of dengue. Medical Journal Armed Forces India. 2013; **69**: 246-253.

[51] Chen Z, Liao Y, Ke X, Zhou J, Chen Y, Gao L, Chen Q, Yu S. Comparison of reverse transcription loop-mediated isothermal amplification, conventional PCR and real-time PCR assays for Japanese encephalitis virus. Molecular Biology Reports. 2011; **38**: 4063-4070.

[52] Li S, Fang M, Zhou B, Ni H, Shen Q, Zhang H, Han Y, Yin J, Chang W, Xu G, Cao G. Simultaneous detection and differentiation of dengue virus serotypes 1-4, Japanese encephalitis virus, and West Nile virus by a combined reverse-transcription loop-mediated isothermal amplification assay. Virology Journal. 2011; **8**: 360.

[53] Teoh B-T, Sam S-S, Tan K-K, Johari J, Danlami MB, Hooi P-S, Md-Esa R, AbuBakar S. Detection of dengue viruses using reverse transcription-loop-mediated isothermal amplification. BMC Infectious Diseases. 2013; **13**: 387.

[54] Couvelard A, Marianneau P, Bedel C, Drouet M-T, Vachon F, Hénin D, Deubel V. Report of a fatal case of dengue infection with hepatitis: demonstration of dengue antigens in hepatocytes and liver apoptosis. Human Pathology. 1999; **30**: 1106-1110.

[55] Balsitis SJ, Coloma J, Castro G, Alava A, Flores D, McKerrow JH, Beatty PR, Harris E. Tropism of dengue virus in mice and humans defined by viral nonstructural protein 3-specific immunostaining. American Journal of Tropical Medicine and Hygiene. 2009; **80**: 416-424.

[56] Nakao S, Lai C-J, Young NS. Dengue virus, a flavivirus, propagates in human bone marrow progenitors and hematopoietic cell lines. Blood. 1989; **74**: 1235-1240.

[57] Cuzzubbo AJ, Endy TP, Nisalak A, Kalayanarooj S, Vaughn DW, Ogata SA, Clements DE, Devine PL. Use of recombinant envelope proteins for serological diagnosis of Dengue virus infection in an immunochromatographic assay. Clinical and Diagnostic Laboratory Immunology. 2001; **8**: 1150-1155.

[58] Kumarasamy V, Wahab AH, Chua SK, Hassan Z, Chem YK, Mohamad M, Chua KB. Evaluation of a commercial dengue NS1 antigen-capture ELISA for laboratory diagnosis of acute dengue virus infection. Journal of Virological Methods. 2007; **140**: 75-79.

[59] Gowri Sankar S, Dhananjeyan KJ, Paramasivan R, Thenmozhi V, Tyagi BK, John Vennison S. Evaluation and use of NS1 IgM antibody detection for acute dengue virus diagnosis: report from an outbreak investigation. Clinical Microbiology and Infection. 2012; **18**: E8–E10.

[60] Young PR, Hilditch PA, Bletchly C, Halloran W. An antigen capture enzyme-linked immunosorbent assay reveals high levels of the dengue virus protein NS1 in the sera of infected patients. Journal of Clinical Microbiology. 2000; **38**: 1053-1057.

[61] Sanyal S, Taylor-Robinson A. Host-virus interactions in dengue infection indicate targets for detection and therapeutic interventions. Immunity and Diseases. 2013; **1**: a7.

[62] Dussart P, Labeau B, Lagathu G, Louis P, Nunes MR, Rodrigues SG, Storck-Herrmann C, Cesaire R, Morvan J, Flamand M, Baril L. Evaluation of an enzyme immunoassay for detection of dengue virus NS1 antigen in human serum. Clinical and Vaccine Immunology. 2006; **13**: 1185-1189.

[63] Bessoff K, Delorey M, Sun W, Hunsperger E. Comparison of two commercially available dengue virus (DENV) NS1 capture enzyme-linked immunosorbent assays using a single clinical sample for diagnosis of acute DENV infection. Clinical and Vaccine Immunology. 2008; **15**: 1513-1518.

[64] Guzmán MG, Jaenisch T, Gaczkowski R, Hang VTT, Sekaran SD, Kroeger A, Vazquez S, Ruiz D, Martinez E, Mercado JC, Balmaseda A, Harris E, Dimano E, Leano PS, Yoksan S, Villegas E, Benduzu H, Villalobos I, Farrar J, Simmons CP. Multi-country evaluation of the sensitivity and specificity of two commercially-available NS1 ELISA assays for dengue diagnosis. PLoS Neglected Tropical Diseases. 2010; **4**: e811.

[65] Ding X, Hu D, Chen Y, Di B, Jin J, Pan Y, Qiu L, Wang Y, Wen K, Wang M, Che X. Full serotype- and group-specific NS1 capture enzyme-linked immunosorbent assay for rapid differential diagnosis of dengue virus infection. Clinical and Vaccine Immunology. 2011; **18**: 430-434.

[66] Xu H, Di B, Pan Y-X, Qiu L-W, Hao W, He L-J, Yuen K-Y, Che X-Y. Serotype 1-specific monoclonal antibody-based antigen capture immunoassay for detection of circulating nonstructural protein NS1: implications for early diagnosis and serotyping of dengue virus infections. Journal of Clinical Microbiology. 2006; **44**: 2872-2878.

[67] Libraty DH, Young PR, Pickering D, Endy TP, Kalayanarooj S, Green S, Vaughn DW, Nisalak A, Ennis FA, Rothman AL. High circulating levels of the dengue virus nonstructural protein NS1 early in dengue illness correlate with the development of dengue hemorrhagic fever. Journal of Infectious Diseases. 2002; **186**: 1165-1168.

[68] Kassim FM, Izati MN, TgRogayah TA, Apandi YM, Saat Z. Use of dengue NS1 antigen for early diagnosis of dengue virus infection. Southeast Asian Journal of Tropical Medicine and Public Health. 2011; **42**: 562-569.

[69] Blacksell SD, Jarman RG, Gibbons RV, Tanganuchitcharnchai A, Mammen MP Jr, Nisalak A, Kalayanarooj S, Bailey MS, Premaratna R, de Silva HJ, Day NP, Lalloo DG. Comparison of seven commercial antigen and antibody enzyme-linked immunosorbent assays for detection of acute dengue infection. Clinical and Vaccine Immunology. 2012; **19**: 804-810.

[70] Osorio L, Ramirez M, Bonelo A, Villar LA, Parra B. Comparison of the diagnostic accuracy of commercial NS1-based diagnostic tests for early dengue infection. Virology Journal. 2010; **7**: 361.

[71] Bollati M, Alvarez K, Assenberg R, Baronti C, Canard B, Cook S, Coutard B, Decroly E, de Lamballerie X, Gould EA, Grard G, Grimes JM, Hilgenfeld R, Jansson AM, Malet H, Mancini EJ, Mastrangelo E, Mattevi A, Milani M, Moureau G, Neyts J, Owens RJ, Ren J, Selisko B, Speroni S, Steuber H, Stuart DI, Unge T, Bolognesi M. Structure and functionality in flavivirus NS-proteins: perspectives for drug design. Antiviral Research. 2010; **87**: 125-148.

[72] Wong SJ, Boyle RH, Demarest VL, Woodmansee AN, Kramer LD, Li H, Drebot M, Koski RA, Fikrig E, Martin DA, Shi PY. Immunoassay targeting nonstructural protein 5 to differentiate West Nile virus infection from dengue and St. Louis encephalitis virus infections and from flavivirus vaccination. Journal of Clinical Microbiology. 2003; **41**: 4217-4223.

[73] Kuno G, Cropp CB, Wong-Lee J, Gubler DJ. Evaluation of an IgM immunoblot kit for dengue diagnosis. American Journal of Tropical Medicine and Hygiene. 1998; **59**: 757-762.

[74] Nimmannitya S, Gubler D, Kuno G. Dengue hemorrhagic fever: diagnosis and management. In: Gubler DJ, Kuno G, editors. Dengue and Dengue Hemorrhagic Fever. Oxford: CAB International; 1997. pp. 133-145.

[75] Thein S, Aaskov J, Myint TT, Shwe TN, Saw TT, Zaw A. Changes in levels of anti-dengue virus IgG subclasses in patients with disease of varying severity. Journal of Medical Virology. 1993; **40**: 102-106.

[76] Koraka P, Suharti C, Setiati TE, Mairuhu AT, Van Gorp E, Hack CE, Juffrie M, Sutaryo J, Van Der Meer GM, Groen J, Osterhaus AD. Kinetics of dengue virus-specific serum immunoglobulin classes and subclasses correlate with clinical outcome of infection. Journal of Clinical Microbiology. 2001; **39**: 4332-4338.

[77] Kao C-L, King C-C, Chao D-Y, Wu H-L, Chang GJ. Laboratory diagnosis of dengue virus infection: current and future perspectives in clinical diagnosis and public health. Journal of Microbiology, Immunology and Infection. 2005; **38**: 5-16.

[78] Clarke DH, Casals J. Techniques for hemagglutination and hemagglutination-inhibition with arthropod-borne viruses. American Journal of Tropical Medicine and Hygiene. 1958; **7**: 561-573.

[79] Subedi D, Taylor-Robinson AW. Laboratory diagnosis of dengue infection: current techniques and future strategies. Open Journal of Clinical Diagnostics. 2014; **4**: 63-70.

[80] Bundo K, Igarashi A. Antibody-capture ELISA for detection of immunoglobulin M antibodies in sera from Japanese encephalitis and dengue hemorrhagic fever patients. Journal of Virological Methods. 1985; **11**: 15-22.

[81] Groen J, Koraka P, Velzing J, Copra C, Osterhaus AD. Evaluation of six immunoassays for detection of dengue virus-specific immunoglobulin M and G antibodies. Clinical and Diagnostic Laboratory Immunology. 2000; **7**: 867-871.

[82] Nepal HP, Ansari S, Gyawali N, Gautam R, Paudel R, Shrestha S, Rimal B, Acharya A, Chapagain ML, Taylor-Robinson AW. Detection of IgM against dengue virus in clinically suspected patients presenting at a tertiary care centre, Narayani Zone, Nepal. Journal of Tropical Diseases & Public Health. 2014; **2**: 139.

[83] Sa-ngasang A, Wibulwattanakij S, Chanama S, O-rapinpatipat A, A-nuegoonpipat A, Anantapreecha S, Sawanpanyalert P, Kurane I. Evaluation of RT-PCR as a tool for diagnosis of secondary dengue virus infection. Japanese Journal of Infectious Diseases. 2003; **56**: 205-209.

[84] World Health Organization. Dengue Haemorrhagic Fever: Diagnosis, Treatment, Prevention and Control. 2nd ed. Geneva: WHO; 1997. 92 p.

[85] Cardosa MJ, Wang SM, Sum MS, Tio PH. Antibodies against prM protein distinguish between previous infection with dengue and Japanese encephalitis viruses. BMC Microbiology. 2002; **2**: 9.

[86] de Souza VAUF, Fernandes S, Araújo ES, Tateno AF, Oliveira OM, dos Reis Oliveira R, Pannuti CS. Use of an immunoglobulin G avidity test to discriminate between primary and secondary dengue virus infections. Journal of Clinical Microbiology. 2004; **42**: 1782-1784.

[87] Matheus S, Deparis X, Labeau B, Lelarge J, Morvan J, Dussart P. Discrimination between primary and secondary dengue virus infection by an immunoglobulin G avidity test using a single acute-phase serum sample. Journal of Clinical Microbiology. 2005; **43**: 2793-2797.

[88] Prince HE, Yeh C, Lapé-Nixon M. Utility of IgM/IgG ratio and IgG avidity for distinguishing primary and secondary dengue virus infections using sera collected more than 30 days after disease onset. Clinical and Vaccine Immunology. 2011; **18**: 1951-1956.

[89] Vaughn DW, Nisalak A, Kalayanarooj S, Solomon T, Dung NM, Cuzzubbo A, Devine PL. Evaluation of a rapid immunochromatographic test for diagnosis of dengue virus infection. Journal of Clinical Microbiology. 1998; **36**: 234-238.

[90] Vajpayee M, Singh UB, Seth P, Broor S. Comparative evaluation of various commercial assays for diagnosis of dengue fever. Southeast Asian Journal of Tropical Medicine and Public Health. 2001; **32**: 472-475.

[91] Kittigul L, Suankeow K. Use of a rapid immunochromatographic test for early diagnosis of dengue virus infection. European Journal of Clinical Microbiology and Infectious Diseases. 2002; **21**: 224-226.

[92] Blacksell SD, Newton PN, Bell D, Kelley J, Mammen MP Jr, Vaughn DW, Wuthiekanun V, Sungkakum A, Nisalak A, Day NP. The comparative accuracy of 8 commercial rapid immunochromatographic assays for the diagnosis of acute dengue virus infection. Clinical Infectious Diseases. 2006; **42**: 1127-1134.

[93] Kalyani D, Bai MM. Evaluation of immunochromatographic test in early serological diagnosis of dengue fever. Indian Journal of Pathology & Microbiology. 2012; **55**: 610-611.

[94] Fry SR, Meyer M, Semple MG, Simmons CP, Sekaran SD, Huang JX, McElnea C, Huang C-Y, Valks A, Young PR, Cooper MA. The diagnostic sensitivity of dengue rapid test assays is significantly enhanced by using a combined antigen and antibody testing approach. PLoS Neglected Tropical Diseases. 2011; **5**: e1199.

[95] Fatima Z, Idrees M, Bajwa MA, Tahir Z, Ullah O, Zia MQ, Hussain A, Akram M, Khubaib B, Afzal S., Munir S, Saleem S, Rauff B, Badar S, Naudhani M, Butt S, Aftab M, Ali L, Ali M. Serotype and genotype analysis of dengue virus by sequencing followed by phylogenetic analysis using samples from three mini outbreaks-2007-2009 in Pakistan. BMC Microbiology. 2011; **11**: 200.

[96] Chakravarti A, Chauhan MS, Kumar S, Ashraf A. Genotypic characterization of dengue virus strains circulating during 2007-2009 in New Delhi. Archives of Virology. 2013; **158**: 571-581.

[97] Ferraz FO, Bomfim MR, Totola AH, Ávila TV, Cisalpino D, Pessanha JE, da Glória de Souza D, Teixeira Júnior AL, Nogueira ML, Bruna-Romero O, Teixeira MM. Evaluation of laboratory tests for dengue diagnosis in clinical specimens from consecutive patients with suspected dengue in Belo Horizonte, Brazil. Journal of Clinical Virology. 2013; **58**: 41-46.

[98] McClure WF. 204 years of near infrared technology: 1800-2003. Journal of Near Infrared Spectroscopy. 2003; **11**: 487-518.

[99] Baeumner AJ, Schlesinger NA, Slutzki NS, Romano J, Lee EM, Montagna RA. Biosensor for dengue virus detection: sensitive, rapid, and serotype specific. Analytical Chemistry. 2002; **74**: 1442-1448.

[100] Zhang G-J, Zhang L, Huang MJ, Luo ZHH, Tay GKI, Lim E-JA, Kang TG, Chen Y. Silicon nanowire biosensor for highly sensitive and rapid detection of Dengue virus. Sensors and Actuators B: Chemical. 2010; **146**: 138-144.

Chapter 5

Optical Diagnostic of Dengue Virus Infected Human Blood using Raman, Polarimetric and Fluorescence Spectroscopy

Shamaraz Firdous and Shahzad Anwar

Additional information is available at the end of the chapter

http://dx.doi.org/10.5772/67954

Abstract

In this chapter, we present the optical diagnosis of normal and dengue viral-infected human blood using Raman, Polarimetric, Transmission, and Fluorescence Spectroscopic techniques. The possibility of using light in diagnosis and treating illness has been known for thousands of years. The properties of light and lasers provided many modern applications at home, in industry, and in the field of medicine. Laser use in the field of medicine is large and steadily growing. This growth is based on the versatility of laser light. Efficient and accurate diagnosis of dengue is of primary importance for clinical care. A range of laboratory diagnostic methods has been developed to support patient management and disease control. The choice of diagnostic method depends on the purpose for which the testing is done, the type of laboratory facilities and technical expertise available, costs, and the time of sample collection. The dengue viral infection is mostly diagnosed through laboratory tests; these tests include detection of the virus, virus antigen, anti-dengue virus antibody, complement fixation test, neutralization tests, and detection of virus nucleic acid. As dengue infection most rapidly increases in different regions, early diagnostic confirmation of dengue infection in patients allows for timely clinical intervention, etiological investigation, and disease control. Hence, diagnosis of dengue disease during the acute phase should be a priority and is a public health concern. Lasers and optics have many applications in medical sciences; diagnosis and treatment of diseases with lasers and light are latest and noninvasive techniques. Development of light-based apparatus has evolved into tools for improved diagnosis and treatment modalities in medical sciences. The methods of the laser spectroscopy make it possible to obtain direct information regarding the structure and dynamics of the functional groups of biomolecules. Development of new light sources, optics, and diode laser of different wavelengths makes them attractive for spectroscopy of biological molecules. In our study, more than 600 dengue viral-infected blood or blood sera samples and 25 non-dengue healthy blood samples were analyzed using four different optical methodologies. In the first study, Raman spectrum peaks for normal samples observed at 1527, 1170, and 1021 cm^{-1} show the presence of different biological materials, including lipids, carbohydrates, skeletal C–C stretch of acyl chains, and guanine. Raman peaks at 1467, 1316, 1083, and 860 cm^{-1} were observed in dengue-infected patients, representing CH2/CH3 deformation of lipids and collagen, guanine, lipids, and protein peaks using 532 nm laser sources. In our second study, an optical diagnosis of dengue virus infection in the whole blood is presented utilizing Mueller matrix polarimetry. Mueller matrices were extracted using light source from 500 to 700 nm with scanning step of 10 nm. Polar decomposition of the Mueller matrices for all the blood samples was performed that yielded polarization properties including depolarization, diattenuation, degree of polarization, retardance and optical activity, out of which, depolarization index clusters up the diseased and healthy into different groups. The average depolarized light in the case of dengue infection in the whole blood decreases, whereas for the healthy blood samples it increased. This suggests that the depolarization index of the polarized light was at wavelengths 500–700 nm; in this case, we find that depolarization index values are higher for dengue viral infection when compared to normal samples. This technique can effectively be used for the characterization of the dengue virus infected at an early stage of the disease. In the third experiment, the transmission absorption spectra of dengue-infected whole blood samples were observed in ultraviolet to near infrared range (400–800 nm) of about 30 conformed infected patients and were compared to normal blood samples. Transmitted spectra of dengue-infected blood showed two strong spectrum peaks at 540 and 580 nm wavelength of illuminating light, whereas in case of normal blood below 600 nm total attenuation was observed. The two strong absorption peaks from 500 to 600 nm are characteristic of cell damage and dengue virus antibodies IgG and IgM produced against dengue antigen. In the last study, we report an optical diagnosis of dengue-infected whole blood and controlled samples with Laser Scanning Confocal Microscopy (LSCM) over a laser excitation of 488, 543, and 633 nm wavelength. Based on our findings, the system has potential applications in the detection and quantification of dengue virus-infected cells, antigen, and antibodies in blood in vitro.

Keywords: optical diagnosis, dengue viral infection, transmission Raman spectroscopy, polarimetry, confocal laser scanning microscopy (CLSM)

1. Introduction

Dengue is an endemic viral disease affecting tropical and subtropical regions around the world and is a viral infection transmitted by the bite of an infected female Aedes mosquito. There are four distinct serotypes of the dengue virus (DEN 1, DEN 2, DEN 3, and DEN 4). Symptoms appear in the first 15 days after the infection. Dengue virus affects humans from newborn baby to aged persons, mostly children and young ones. Dengue fever has no treatment yet, but precautions, early diagnoses, and proper care can protect patients from severity [1–4]. Recently, most of dengue viral infection cases are from Asia, Europe, Africa, and even America. Last year, majority of cases were from Asia and Africa. In 2013, indigenous transmission of dengue was also reported in America and Europe. Dengue spread in America and Europe is mostly by the movement of infected persons and goods; the lack of healthy environment and preventive arrangements also contribute to the global increase of dengue [5–7].

The World Health Organization estimates that worldwide each year, there may be approximately 100 million cases of dengue virus infections [8, 9]. Dengue spread is mostly related with special kind of mosquito bites; however, some normal mosquitoes are infected through dengue virus and then become the source of infection. Dengue virus spreads from person to person but not directly. In fact, it can never transfer from one person to another directly [10, 11].

An evaluation of commercial capture immunosorbent assay for detection of immunoglobulin M and G antibodies produced during dengue infection and Pan Bio kit was evaluated with paired serum specimens from patients. They proved that ELISA should be useful in the clinical diagnosis of dengue infection. Similarly, an evaluation of a commercial ELISA kit for the detection of IgM during dengue infection revealed that primary dengue infection was detected positive for anti-dengue antibodies. Study of Pan Bio duo ELISA and MRL dengue fever IgM capture ELISA for the diagnosis of dengue virus infection in Southeast Asia was done, and comparing the specificity and sensitivity of the tests at different cutoff values revealed that similarly in distinguishing dengue virus from non-flaviviruses showed significantly better distinction between dengue virus and other viruses [12]. Dengue-infected person generates antibodies against dengue virus, which cannot be observed in normal blood or blood sera. The optical changes observed are reflection of biochemical changes in blood. This is the basic principle of dengue fever diagnosis based on optical spectroscopic techniques [13].

Medical tools and sensors based on lasers and optics are used in many applications. Optical diagnostic apparatus are very effective as compared to conventional disease detection methods. Optical techniques are noninvasive, direct, cost-effective, and easy to use with high specificity, sensitivity, and small size. Optical diseases diagnostic research and development has been useful to healthcare, environmental applications, biotechnology industry, and medical sciences [14, 15]. For the development of new optical equipment to be used in medical sciences and devices for practical applications, all the experimental findings and practical aspects, such as robustness, reproducibility, simplicity, and shelf life, should be carefully considered. In these experimental results and optical detection of different diseases using light allows construction of sensitive, simple, and cheap analytical devices with a wide variety of possible applications in screening and monitoring of diseases for use in personalized medicine, remote areas or in developing countries where the availability of inexpensive diagnostic tools are not accessible [16, 17].

2. Raman spectroscopy

Raman spectroscopy was carried out using high-resolution Raman spectroscopy system. The main elements of setup are laser sources 532nm, samples slides, and chamber light collection optics detection system. The target material, blood serum of normal, and dengue samples on glass substrate at room temperature (300±2 K) are used as optimized parameters. The sample was excited by He-Cd laser of 532 nm wavelength and 80 mw power, and output intensity signal detected with objective lens and air-cooled charge-coupled device (CCD) detector. The Raman spectra collected in Raman shift of 600–1800 cm^{-1}. We used the accumulate acquisition mode to reduce noise and thermal fluctuation and improve signal to noise ratio [18–20].

For normal blood sera, the Raman shifts are observed at 1527, 1170, and 1023 cm^{-1} with intensity level of 7200–9500 pixels, showing a compound that occurs in guano and fish scales and is one of the four constituent bases of nucleic acids. A pure derivative, it is paired with cytosine in double-stranded DNA (guanine). Adenine is used in forming nucleotides of the nucleic acids. Adenine can be found in DNA and RNA, in first with two hydrogen bonds for the nucleic acid structures stabilization and in second for protein synthesis. Tryptophan is α-amino acid that is used in the biosynthesis of proteins TRP (protein) carbohydrates peak for solids. Carbon skeletons are the backbones of organic molecules. They are composed of carbon-carbon atoms that form chains to make an organic compound. Length, shape, location, and amount of double bonds are characteristics of carbon skeletons (skeletal C-C), and Cardiolipins are a subclass of glycerophospholipids containing four acyl chains and three glycerol groups that are particularly abundant in the inner mitochondrial membrane. They are believed to activate enzymes involved with oxidative phosphorylation (stretch of lipids acyl chains) as shown in **Figure 1A**. The Raman shifts observed in Raman spectrum of a dengue-infected blood serum are at 1467, 1316, 1083, and 860 cm^{-1} with intensity level of 6000–7500 pixels attributed to the bands of stretching and deformation vibrations of CH_2, C-CH_3, and OCH_3 groups in the infrared and Raman spectra (CH_2/CH_3) deformation of lipids and collagen, guanine, lipids, and protein bands as shown in **Figure 1B**.

The main dengue viral infection sera peaks appear at 1467 and 860 cm^{-1}. The intensity of these peaks, as well as those at 1316 and 1081 cm^{-1}, is plotted against the intensity level in **Figure 1B**. In our previous chapter [6], we reported transmission spectra of dengue-infected whole blood samples irradiated with light of 400–800 nm wavelength. We collected data of 30 conformed infected patients and compared them to normal blood samples. Transmission spectra of dengue-infected blood show strong and prominent peaks at 540 and 580 nm. In case of normal blood, total absorption has been observed from 400 to 600 nm of wavelength. In case of dengue, the peaks indicate damage and dengue virus antibodies immunoglobulin G (IgG) and immunoglobulin M (IgM) produced against dengue antigen. In another chapter, we determined that normal whole blood and serum characteristic peaks were excited at 442 and 532 nm. In dengue-infected whole blood and serum, two peaks at 1614 and 1750 cm^{-1} are observed, which are due to the presence of immunoglobulin antibodies IgG and IgM.

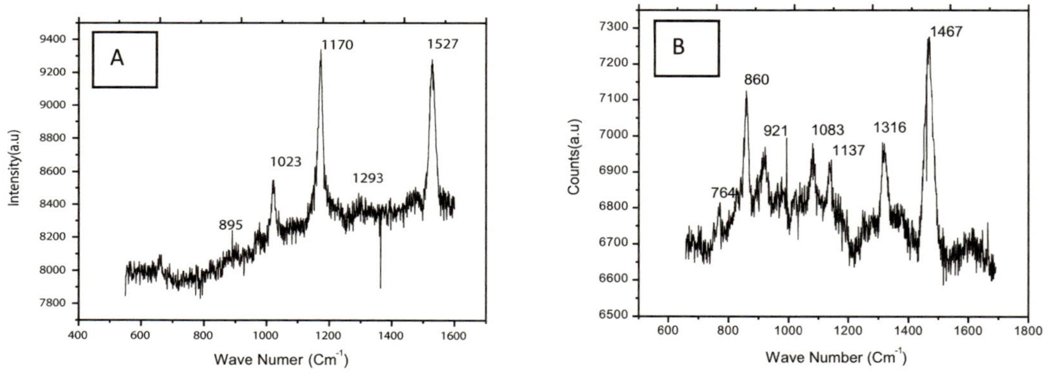

Figure 1. Raman spectrum of (A) normal blood and (B) dengue blood at 532nm wavelength of light.

http://dx.doi.org/10.5772/67954

Raman spectroscopy has proven to be an effective analytical approach in geology, semiconductor, materials, and polymer science fields. The application of Raman spectroscopy and microscopy within biology is rapidly increasing because it can provide chemical and compositional information. Raman spectroscopic technique based on protein and lipid changes due to antibodies and antigen reactions, while the Protein and lipids concentration totally changes in dengue viral sample as compared to normal ones [21].

3. Mueller matrix polarimetry

Polarimeters are optical instruments used for determining the polarization properties of light beams and samples. To perform accurate polarimetry, all the issues necessary for careful and accurate radiometry must be considered together with many additional polarization issues. Mueller matrix polarimetry yields four optical parameters, namely depolarization coefficient, linear retardance, optical activity, and diattenuation, which can be used to characterize the tissues or turbid media [22–34]. We represented very interesting results from the dengue-infected whole blood by exploiting the depolarization nature of polarized light in whole blood; this can be used for the discrimination between the healthy and viral infection diseased blood samples [5].

Mueller matrices from all the 30 ultra-thin smeared blood slides were acquired using Mueller Matrix Polarimeter AxoScan™ (Axometrics, USA). AxoScan™ system employs dual rotating retarder as discussed in our previous study [5]. A tunable light source ranging from 400 to 800 nm, coupled with 200 nm multimode fiber optic probe, is used to shine the sample through Polarization State Generator (PSG). Light source consists of a low-noise 150 W Xenon arc lamp and a scanning diffraction-grating monochromatic light. PSG consists of a fixed linear polarizer along with a rotating linear retarder. As the retarder rotates, a wide variety of polarization states, including linear (horizontal, vertical), elliptical (−45°/+45°), and circular (left/right),is generated. These six polarization states are steered to pass through the smeared blood slides. The rotating retarder in PSG is rotated five times faster than the retarder in the generator for different combinations of the rotation angles of retarders in PSG and Polarization State Analyzer (PSA); light coming out from PSA is collected by a very sensitive detector. The resulting combination of polarization states at different rotation angles of retarders in PSG and PSA is adequate for determining the Mueller matrix of the sample.

In the present study, Mueller matrices from all the blood samples were measured from 500 to 800 nm, and their polar decomposition yields the polarization parameters for each wavelength, out of which depolarization coefficients showed distinct differentiation. **Figures 2** and **3** displayed the diattenuation and retardance of the dengue-infected and non-dengue healthy blood samples as a function of wavelength. We find that in the case of dengue viral infection, diattenuation and retardance values are lower when compared to normal samples. The diattenuation and retardance of both types of samples can be used for the characterization of the early stage detection of dengue infection in the human blood. The Mueller matrix is generally a diagonal matrix having $m_{00}= 1$ and $m_{11}= m_{22}$. The $m_{11}= m_{22}$ is due to axial symmetry of the material.

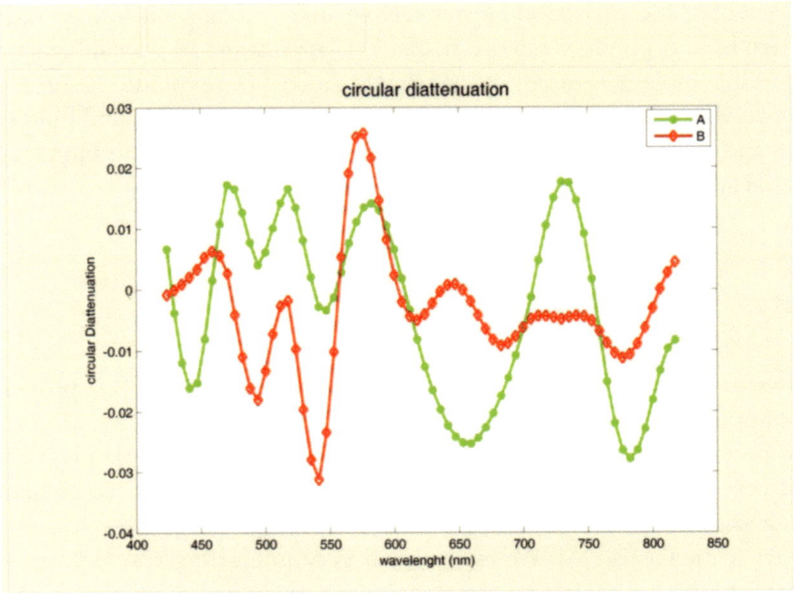

Figure 2. Polarization properties in terms of Mueller matrix, diattenuation of normal (—●—), and of dengue-infected blood (—◆—) at 400–800nm wavelength.

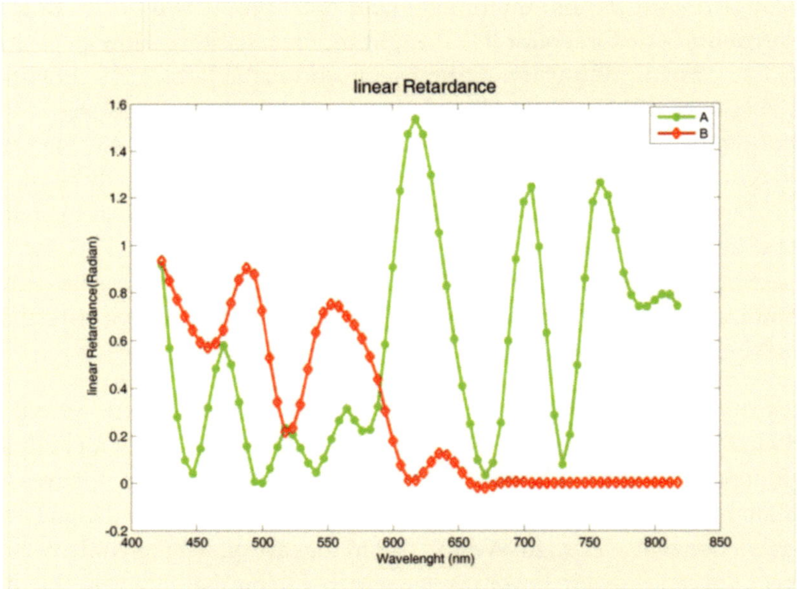

Figure 3. Polarization properties in terms of Mueller matrix, retardance of normal (—●—), and of dengue-infected blood (—◆—) at 400–800nm wavelength.

The retardance matrix is also a diagonal matrix, where all diagonal elements are equal as shown in **Figure 4**. The optical characteristics of dengue-infected samples at 540 nm of light showing depolarization index values were higher as compared to normal samples. The diattenuation is less than polarization as seen in the first row and first column of the Mueller matrix. In the retardance matrix, image m_{11} and m_{22} are same. m_{33} depends on the size of scatterers.

The color intensity of the elements m_{11}, m_{22}, and m_{33} increases when compared to the retardance image of **Figure 4** of dengue-infected ones. The depolarization image is showing a diagonal matrix with maximum intensity at diagonal elements. It is clear that depolarization coefficient decreases as a function of wavelength for both types of samples, as well as the difference of depolarization coefficients reduces for both types of the samples. The hematocrit of the dengue virus-infected blood increases due to decreasing platelets; this increasing of volume fraction of red blood cells may be responsible for the more depolarization coefficient in comparison with the non-dengue healthy blood samples as red blood cells play an important role in scattering that causes the depolarization of polarized light.

In the dengue virus-infected human blood, antibodies IgM and IgG appeared against the infection by the defensive system. These antibodies are like protein structures that must also be responsible for producing more depolarization effects in the dengue-infected blood samples.

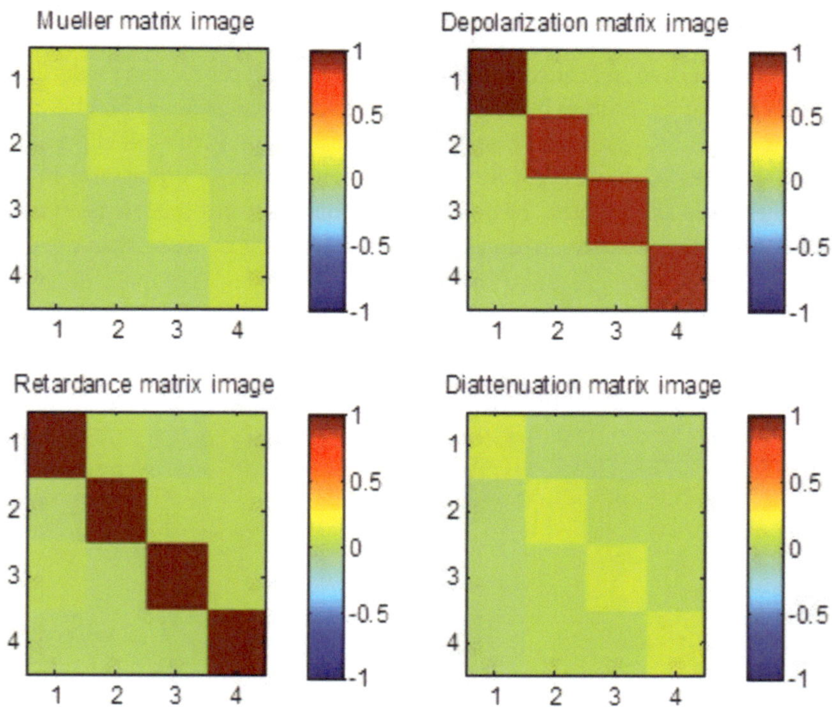

Figure 4. Polarization properties in terms of Mueller matrix, depolarization, retardance, and diattenuation matrix of dengue-infected blood at 540 nm of light.

Mueller matrix polarimetry has been exploited successfully for the optical diagnosis of dengue virus infection in human blood. Depolarization coefficient of the dengue-infected and non-dengue human blood samples is clearly distinct in light spectra for the characterization of both types of samples. In addition, diattenuation, retardance, and depolarization coefficients may be helpful for monitoring the disease from time to time and to monitor very minute structural changes in the tissue of blood chemistry.

4. Transmission spectroscopy

In this study, we provide transmission spectroscopy of dengue viral infection analysis. The cell culture method is still considered the standard for viral diagnosis as it has the advantages of detecting infectious viral particles and the ability to achieve low detection limits. This new method has the potential to be extended for the detection of other viruses and adapted into a portable, automated system for detection of viruses from environmental samples. The presented results are very effective for initial screening of dengue-infected patients and to minimize the diagnostic cost [6].

We used Avaspec. Spectrometer (Avantes Inc, Netherlands) of wavelength range 400–1000 nm and Avaspec.software to record data. About 50 μl drop of whole blood excited with light as shown in **Figure 5**. Two prominent absorption peaks at 540 and 580 nm of blood spectrum, as measured within a set of about 30 essentially conformed dengue-infected individuals, are observed as shown in **Figure 6**. The change represented by these peaks in the protein and blood cells within the human body is a manifestation of significant biochemical changes due to the antibodies IgG activated after 2–3 days of dengue virus infection and IgM produced after one week. We have recorded transmission spectra of other viral-infected blood samples, like hepatitis and malaria, besides dengue infection, but there is no transmission in the range of 400–600 nm. The spectrum peaks at 540 and 580 nm are only in dengue-infected samples.

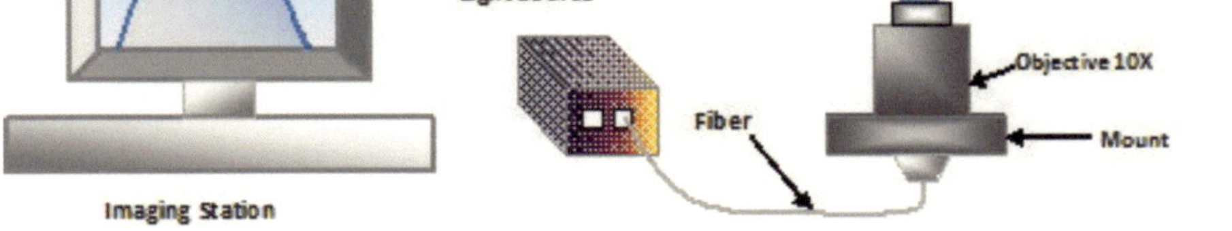

Figure 5. Experimental setup for the whole blood dengue infection diagnosis with light spectroscopy.

http://dx.doi.org/10.5772/67954

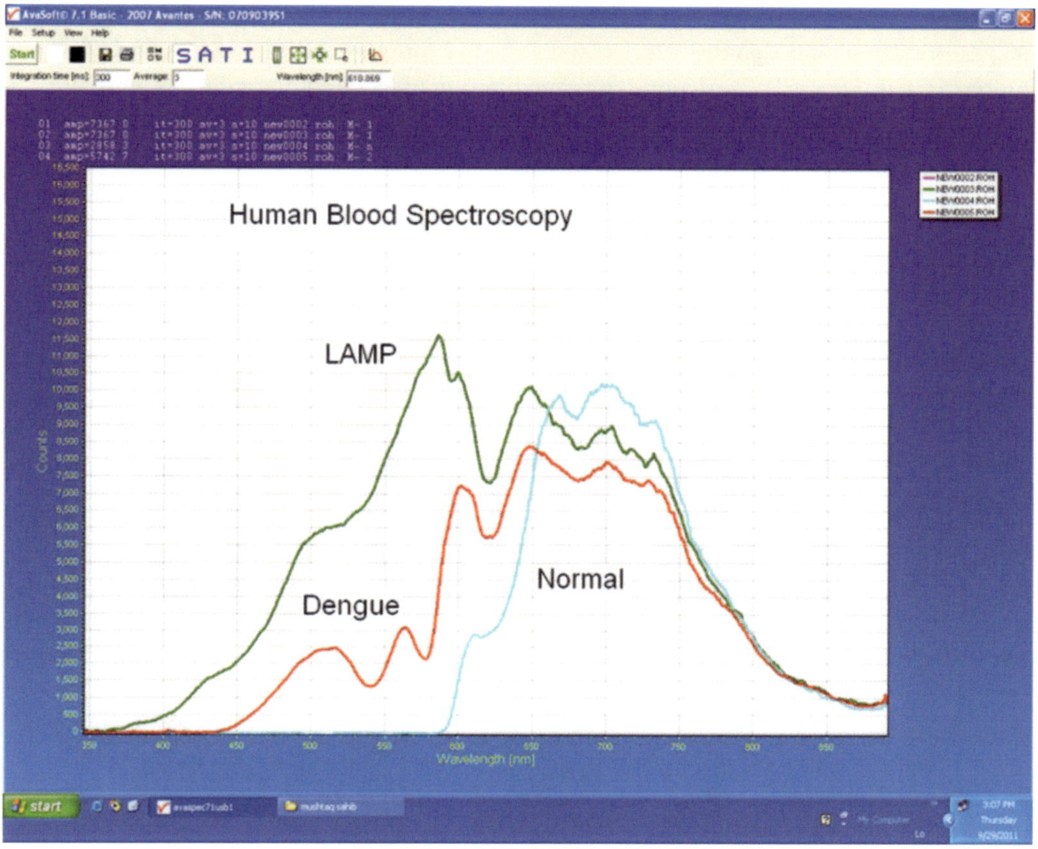

Figure 6. The transmission spectroscopy of normal and dengue-infected whole blood spectrum at 400–1000 nm wavelength.

5. Confocal microscopic analysis

We have used light spectroscopy, Raman and absorption spectroscopy, and Laser scanning confocal microscopy (LSCM) techniques for repaid screening of dengue infection. LSCM has become an invaluable tool for a wide range of investigations in the biological and medical sciences for imaging thin optical sections in living and fixed specimens. To image the dengue-infected blood, a drop of 50μl whole blood was placed on quartz glass slide and seen through (63X, 100X) water and oil emulsions objectives of LSCM (LSM-510, Carl Zeiss, Micro Imaging Inc., Germany) equipped with 451, 471, 488, and 517nm line of Argon ion, 553 and 633 nm He-Ne lasers, 10 to 100X water and oil emulsions objectives and three Photo Multiplier Tubes (PMTs). Fluorescence light from the sample was collected by the objective, directed to an analyzer, and spatially filtered by the confocal pinhole in the detection path. Reflected light that passed through the pinhole was spectrally separated by dichroic filters and directed to three PMTs to detect light at each wavelength. Images were acquired as 8-bit TIFF files (512 × 512 pixel frame) and processed using Zen software (Carl Zeiss, Micro Imaging Inc., Germany).

We demonstrated the dengue-infected human blood in in vitro using LSCM. The confocal images of normal and dengue-infected whole blood samples are analyzed with LSCM and fluorescence is detected. The dengue cells are different in looks compared to the normal ones, and the fluorescence from dengue infected is prominent than normal as shown in **Figure 7**. The whole blood analyzed on day 10 and day 13 shows antibodies IgG and IgM structure over blood cells. We suggest that as platelets decrease, fluorescence increase due to complex interactions between the virus and host cells, leading to the activation of transcription factors, cytokines, and enzymatic factors. The simple blood images taken at day 3 of infection are shown in **Figure 7** and fluorescence of cells at day 10 is shown in **Figure 8**. These interactions may induce not only pathologic prion flammatory responses that influence the severity and progression of the disease but also virus clearance and apoptotic pathways that could be controlling infection by anti-viral mechanisms. The present study may, therefore, contribute to a better understanding of the cell activation mechanisms triggered during dengue infections occurring in human target cells. The viral infection images at day 10 and 13 after infection are shown in **Figure 8**.

Blood sample analysis with LSCM provides a way for diagnosis of infection. The results obtained can be used in the development of new methods and optimization of existing ones for dengue-infected patients. The presented techniques can be used for new light-based diagnostic apparatus for the quantities analysis of dengue patients. In our previous research findings,

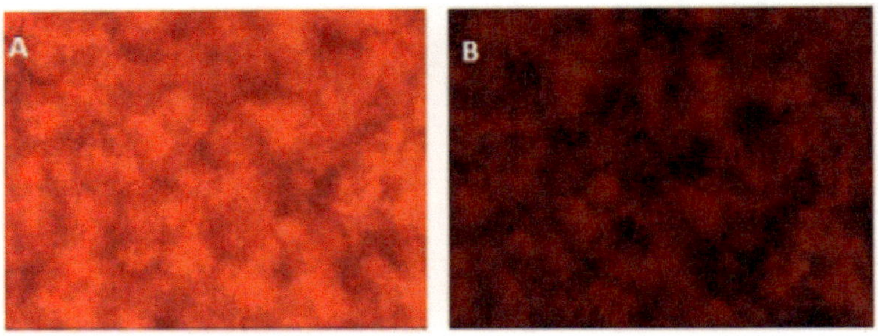

Figure 7. An early comparison of dengue-infected blood samples with a confocal microscope (63×). (A) normal blood drop on glass slide and (B) dengue-infected blood at day 4 after infection.

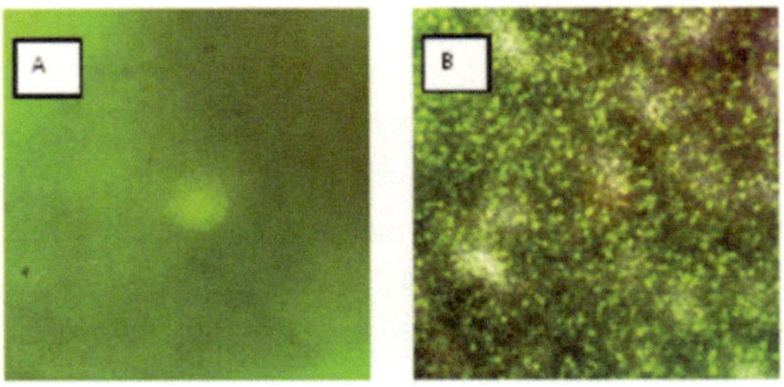

Figure 8. An early comparison of dengue-infected blood samples with a confocal microscope (63×). (A) normal blood drop on glass slide and (B) dengue-infected blood at day 10 after infection.

we have characterized tissues and biomaterials for optical imaging to diagnose diseases and develop optical detection equipments [35–53].

Author details

Shamaraz Firdous* and Shahzad Anwar

*Address all correspondence to: shamaraz@gmail.com

Biophotonics Laboratories, National Institute of Lasers and Optronics (NILOP), Islamabad, Pakistan

References

[1] Meinke GM, Helfmann J,Friebel M (2007) Optical properties of platelets and blood plasma and their influence on the optical behavior of whole blood in the visible to near infrared wavelength range. J Biomedical Optics 12(1):14024-14032

[2] Shu PY, Huang HJ (2004) Current advances in dengue diagnosis. Clin Diagn Lab Immunol 11:642-650

[3] Monath TP (1994) Dengue: the risk to developed and developing countries. Proceedings of the National Academy of Sciences of United States of America. 91:395-400

[4] Rehman A, Anwar S, Firdous S, Ahmed M, Rasheed R, Nawaz M (2012) Dengue blood analysis by Raman spectroscopy. Laser Physics 22(6):1085-1089

[5] Shahzad Anwar, Shamaraz Firdous (2016) Optical diagnosis of dengue virus infected human blood using Mueller matrix polarimetry. Opt Spectrosc 121(2):322-325

[6] Firdous S, Ahmed M, Rehman A, Nawaz M, Anwar S, Murtaza S (2012) Transmission spectroscopy of dengue viral infection. Laser Phys Lett 9(4):317-321

[7] Firdous S, Anwar S (2017) Confocal microscopic analysis of dengue infected blood.

[8] Verma SP (1986) Low levels of irradiation modify lipid domains in model membranes: a laser Raman study. Radiation Research 107(2):183-193

[9] World Health Organization (1986) Dengue haemorrhagic fever: diagnosis, treatment and control. Geneva: WHO, pp. 1-58

[10] Chakravarti A, Matlani M, Kashyap B, Kumar A (2012) Awareness of changing trends in epidemiology of dengue fever is essential for epidemiological surveillance. Indian Journal of Medical Microbiology 30:222-226.

[11] Subedi D., Taylor-Robinson AW (2014) Laboratory diagnosis of dengue infection: current techniques and future strategies. Open Journal of Clinical Diagnostics 2014.doi:10.4236/ojcd.2014.41012

[12] Pei-Yun Shu, Jyh-Hsiung Huang (2004) Current advances in dengue diagnosis. Clinical and Laboratory Immunology 11(4) 642-650

[13] Puppels GJ, Garritsen HS, Segers-Nolten GM, de Mul FF, Greve J (1991) Raman microspectroscopic approach to the study of human granulocytes. Biophysical Journal 60(5): 1046-1056

[14] Narayahan S, Galloway L, Nonoyama A, Leparc GF, Garcia LH, Potter RL (2002)UV-visible spectrophotometric approach to blood typing II: phenotyping of subtype A2 and weak D and whole blood analysis.Transfusion42(5):619-626

[15] Lagali NS, Burns NK, Zimmerman D, Munger R (2007) Spectroscopic whole-blood indicators of end-stage renal disease and the hemodialysis treatment. Photochemistry and Photobiology 83(5):1186-1192

[16] O'Faolain E, Hunter MB, Byrne JM, Kelehan P, McNamara M, Byrne HJ, et al (2005) A study examining the effects of tissue processing on human tissue sections using vibrational spectroscopy. Vibrational Spectroscopy 38(1-2):121-127

[17] Krishna CM, Sockalingum GD, Kurien J, Rao L, Venteo L, Pluot M et al (2004) Micro-Raman spectroscopy for optical pathology of oral squamous cell carcinoma. Applied Spectroscopy 58(9):1128-1135

[18] Cafferata ML, Bardach A, Rey-Ares L, Alcaraz A, Cormick G, Gibbons L, Romano M, Cesaroni S, Ruvinsky S (2013) Dengue epidemiology and burden of disease in Latin America and the Caribbean: asystematic review of the literature and meta-analysis. Value in Health Regional Issues 2:347-356

[19] Firdous S, Anwar S, Waheed A, Maraj M (2016) Optical characterization of pure vegetable oils and their biodiesels using Raman spectroscopy. Laser Physics 26(4):045601

[20] S. Anwar, S. Firdous, A. Rehman, and M. Nawaz, Raman Optical Diagnostic of Breast Cancer using Raman, Polarimetric Fluorescence Spectroscopy, Laser phy. Letter 12(4) 045601 (2015).

[21] Shamaraz Firdous, Shahzad Anwar (2015)Dengue viral infection monitoring from diagnostic to recovery using Raman spectroscopy. Laser Physics Letters 12(8):085601

[22] Firdous S, Atif M, Nawaz M(2011) Stokes vector determination of polarized light propagation in turbid medium. Optics and Spectroscopy 110(3):438-441

[23] Firdous S, Hassan K, Ikram M (2005)Formulation of Mueller matrix and modeling of depolarizing and scattering of nitrobenzene in a Kerr Cell. Applied Optics 44(7):1171-1177

[24] Firdous S, Ikram M (2005) Polarized Mueller matrix analytical model for glucose measurement in vitro. Turkish Journal of Medical Science 35:145-159

[25] Firdous S, Atif M, Nawaz M (2010)The optical polarimetric study of blood malignancy in vitro for diagnostic and treatment of blood diseases. Lasers in Engineering 19(5-6):291-305

[26] Firdous S, Fuzail M, Atif M, Nawaz M (2011) Polarimetric characterization of ultra-high molecular weight polyethylene (UHMWPE) for bone substitute biomaterials. Optik 122(2):99-104

[27] Firdous S, Ahmed A, Nawaz M, Ikram M (2013) Optical characterization of chitosan for application as an engineered biomaterial. Optik: International Journal for Light and Electron Optics 124(12):1297-1302

[28] Firdous S, Waqas W, Idrees M, Nawaz M, Ikram M (2013) Polarization sensitive optical imaging of biomaterials using Mueller matrix polarimetric algorithm. Lasers in Engineering 26(3/4):157-180

[29] Ahmed M, Ali S, Mehmood S, Khurshid A, Firdous S, Ikram M (2013) Ex-vivo assessment of carbon tetrachloride(CCL_4) induced chronic injury using polarized light spectroscopy. Applied Spectroscopy 67(12):1382-1389

[30] Aziz T, Firdous S, Rehman T, Khan MA (2013) Polarimetric study of leukemia human peripheral blood smears in 400-800nm spectral range. Optik: International Journal for Light and Electron Optics124(1):2936-2942

[31] Rehman A, Ahmad I, Rehman K, Anwar S, Firdous S, Nawaz M (2015) Optical properties measurement of highly diffusive tissue phantoms for biomedical applications. Laser Physics 25(2):025605

[32] Anwar S, Mubarik M, Waheed A, Firdous S (2015)Polarization imaging and characterization of Chitosan for applications in tissue engineering. Optik:International Journal for Light and Electron Optics 126:871-876

[33] Kamal A, Bashir M, Firdous S, Yasin T, Tariq M, Ikram M, Mehmood MS (2016) Optical properties of ultra-high molecular weight polyethylene (UHMWPE): a material of choice for total joint applications. Radiation Physics and Chemistry118:102-106

[34] Firdous Shamaraz, Anwar Shahzad (2016) Noninvasive optical diagnostic of breast cancer using depolarization of light. Optik 127(5):3035-3038

[35] Rice William, Firdous Shamaraz, Gupta Sharad, Hunter Martin, Foo Cheryl WP, Wang Yongzhong, Kim Hyeon Joo, Kaplan David L, Georgaukodi Irene (2008) Non-invasive characterization of structure and morphology of silk fibroin biomaterials using nonlinear microscopy. Biomaterials 29:2014-2021

[36] Atif M, Firdous S, Khurshid A, Noreen L, Zaidi S, Ikram M (2009) In vitro study of 5 aminolevulinic acid (5-ALA) based photodynamic therapy for apoptosis in human cervical HeLa cell line. Laser Physics Letters 6(12):886-891

[37] Khan Y, Mehmood M, Ahmad J, Riaz Khan M, Firdous S (2010) Low temperature synthesis of fluorescent ZnO nanoparticles. Applied Surface Science 257:1756-1761

[38] Ullah H, Atif M, Firdous S, Mehmood S, Ikram M, Kurachi C, Grecco C, Nicolodelli G, Bagnato VS (2010) Femtosecond light distribution at skin and liver of rats: analysis for use in optical diagnostics. Laser Physics Letters 7-12:889-898

[39] Atif M, Firdous S, Nawaz M (2010) Laser induced effects in different biological samples. Lasers in Medical Sciences 25(4):545-550

[40] Khursid A, Atif M, Firdous S, Zaidi S, Suleman R, Ikram M (2010)Study of the efficacy of 5 ALA_mediated photodynamic therapy of human larynx squamous cell carcinoma (Hep2c) using 5-aminolevulanic acid in vitro. Laser Physics 20(7):1673-1678

[41] Alam F, Roohi S, Atif M, Firdous S, Amir N, Zahoor R (2010) Labelling and optimization of photofrin with ^{99m}Tc. Radiochimica Acta 98:1-6

[42] Atif M, Alam F, Firdous S, Zaidi S, Suleman R, Ikram M. (2010) Study of the efficacy of 5-ALA mediated photodynamic therapy on human rhabdomyosarcoma cell line (RD). Laser Physics Letters 7:757-764

[43] Ullah H, Atif M, Firdous S, Mehmood S, Hamza Y, Imran M, Hussan G, Ikram M. (2011) Optical properties of normal and thermally coagulated chicken liver tissue measured ex vivo with diffuse reflectance. Optics and Spectroscopy 11(2):311-317

[44] Ikram M, Khan R, Firdous S, Atif M, Nawaz M (2011) Photodynamic therapy of non-melanoma skin cancers. Laser Physics 21(2):427-433

[45] Atif M, Firdous S, Mahmood R, Fakhar_e_Alam M, Zaidi SSZ, Suleman R, Ikram M, Nawaz M. Cytotoxic and photocytotoxic effect of photofrin® on human laryngeal carcinoma (Hep2c) cell line. Laser Physics 21(7):1235-1242

[46] Khan RU, Khurshid N, Ikram M, Firdous S, Atif M (2011)Pain during topical photodynamic therapy in Pakistani and Afghani patients. Photodiagnosis and Photodynamic Therapy 8(2):145-146

[47] Fakhar_e_Alam M, Firdous S, Atif M, Khan Y, Zaidi SSZ, Suleman R, Rehman A, Khan RU, Nawaz M, Ikram M (2011) The potential applications of ZnO nanoparticles conjugated with ALA and photofrin as a biomarker in HepG2 cells. Laser Physics 21(11):2156-2154

[48] Fakhar-e-Alam M, Atif M, Rehman T, Sadia H, Firdous S (2011) The role of sensitivity of ALA (PpIX)-based PDT on human embryonic kidney cell line (HEK293T).Laser Physics 21(8):1428-1437

[49] KhurshidA, Firdous S, Ahmat L, Ferraria J, Vollet-Filho JD, Kurachi C, Bagneto VS, Nawaz M, Ikram M, Ahmad M (2012) In vivo study of laser irradiation of fractionated drug administration based mechanism for effective photodynamic therapy in rat liver. Laser Physics 22(1):317-321

[50] Rehman A, Firdous S, Nawaz M, Ahmad M (2012) Optical parameters measurement for diagnostic and photodynamic therapy of human cervical adenocarcinoma (HeLa) cell line. Laser Physics 22(1):322-326

[51] Firdous S, Nawaz M, Ikram M, Ahmed M (2012) In vitro study of cell death with 5-Aminolevulinic acid based photodynamic therapy to improve the efficiency of cancer treatment. Laser Physics 22(3):626-633

[52] Firdous S, Nawaz M, Ahmed M, Anwar S, Rehman A, Rashid R, Mahmood A (2012) Measurement of diabetic sugar concentration in human blood using Raman spectroscopy. Laser Physics 22(6):1-5

[53] Anwar S, Firdous S (2015) Optical diagnostic of Hepatitis B(HBV) and C (HCV) from human blood serum using Raman spectroscopy. Laser Physics Letters 12(7):076001

Section 3

Control Strategies

Chapter 6

Insecticide-Treated House Screens to Reduce Infestations of Dengue Vectors

Pablo Manrique-Saide, Azael Che-Mendoza, Josué Herrera-Bojórquez, Josué Villegas Chim, Guillermo Guillermo-May, Anuar Medina-Barreiro, Felipe Dzul-Manzanilla, Abdiel Martín-Park, Gabriela González-Olvera, Hugo Delfín-Gonzalez, Juan I. Arredondo-Jiménez, Adriana E. Flores-Suarez, Norma Pavía-Ruz, Catrin Huws Jones, Audrey Lenhart and Gonzalo Vazquez-Prokopec

Additional information is available at the end of the chapter

http://dx.doi.org/10.5772/67934

Abstract

The public health importance of the endophilic mosquito *Aedes aegypti* increased dramatically in the recent decade, because it is the vector of dengue, chikungunya, Zika and yellow fever. The use of long-lasting insecticidal nets (LLINs) fixed on doors and windows, as insecticide-treated screening (ITS), is one innovative approach recently evaluated for *Aedes* control in South Mexico. From 2009 to 2014, cluster-randomised controlled trials were conducted in Acapulco and Merida. Intervention clusters received *Aedes*-proof houses ('Casas a prueba de *Aedes*') with ITS and were followed up during 2 years. Overall, results showed significant and sustained reductions on indoor adult vector densities in the treated clusters with ITS after 2 years: ca. 50% on the presence (OR ≤ 0.62, P < 0.05) and abundance (IRR ≤ 0.58, P < 0.05). ITS on doors and windows are 'user-friendly' tool, with high levels of acceptance, requiring little additional work or behavioural change by householders. Factors that favoured these interventions were (a) house construction, (b) high coverage achieved due to the excellent acceptance by the community and (c) collaboration of the vector control services; and only some operational complaints relating to screen fragility and the installation process. ITS is a housing improvement that should be part of the current paradigms for urban vector-borne disease control.

Keywords: *Aedes aegypti*, dengue, chikungunya, Zika, prevention, long-lasting insecticidal nets, insecticide-treated screens, house screening

1. Introduction

Dengue remains a priority for public health authorities across the globe. The viral disease is transmitted primarily by the human-biting mosquito *Aedes aegypti*, which also transmits other viruses, including yellow fever, chikungunya and Zika [1–3]. Although there are several vaccine candidates for dengue, chikungunya and Zika, but none is highly effective. Therefore, preventing or reducing Dengue (DEN) and the transmission of other *Aedes*-borne diseases depend entirely on control of the mosquito vectors or interruption of human-vector contact.

Control of *A. aegypti* is mostly performed in the context of public health and depends on structured programmes sustained by ministries of health. Routine vector control efforts, mostly targeting the outdoor allocation of *Aedes* vectors (i.e. source reduction, hand-applied larvicides to artificial breeding sites and outdoor ultralow volume (ULV) adulticiding), have to date achieved only a limited success in preventing diseases [4]. Improving urban *Aedes* control and achieving a measurable impact on DEN transmission require a reformulation of current strategies and a stronger focus on the adult mosquitoes that actually transmit the disease, both lowering vector abundance and preventing human-vector contact [5, 6].

Females of *A. aegypti* mosquitoes have an endophilic behaviour (within buildings) and methods targeting these locations which have great potential for sustained impact. Methods currently accessible to reduce indoor adult vector abundance and prevent human-vector contact include essentially the control of adult vectors with insecticides (adulticides) applied by institutional programmes either as residual surface treatments or as space treatments; personal protection to reduce exposure to biting with the use of chemical products such as domestic insecticides, repellents and long-lasting insecticidal nets (LLINs) deployed as curtains or bed nets and changes to human habitation or behaviour such as installing mosquito screening on doors, windows and other entry points.

We recently tested in Mexico an innovative intervention called *Aedes aegypti*-proof houses ('Casas a prueba de *Aedes aegypti*' in Spanish), involving insecticide-treated screening (ITS) with LLINs permanently fitted to windows and doors as an innovative approach to exclude *A. aegypti* from houses in dengue endemic areas. Here, we present the results of the evaluation of these ITS-based interventions on the dengue vectors in South Mexico.

2. Long-lasting insecticidal nets (LLINs) for *A. aegypti* control

A LLIN is a factory-produced mosquito netting preloaded with a synthetic pyrethroid insecticide that is intended to retain its biological activity for at least 20 standard washes under laboratory conditions and 3 years of recommended use under field conditions [7]. LLINs, particularly bed nets, are among the most effective approaches for controlling mosquito-borne infections and reducing the global burden of malaria [8] but also can be effective for lymphatic filariasis, Japanese encephalitis and other arboviruses [9].

The use of LLINs is considered a highly effective, safe, affordable, low-tech, long-lasting and simple intervention with effects both at the individual (i.e. bed nets preventing the vector from blood feeding) and community levels (i.e. by reducing the vector lifespan and population).

LLINs are expected to reduce human-vector contact and reduce their life expectancy as a physical barrier, blocking mosquitoes, and as a chemical method, irritating/deterring or eventually killing mosquitoes [10, 11].

Based on the successful control demonstrated against nocturnal endophilic *Anopheles* spp. vectors and protective efficacy of LLINs (in the form of treated bed nets) in reducing malaria transmission [8, 12, 13], the WHO Dengue Scientific Working Group of 2006 identified the development/evaluation of LLINs as a primary global research stream [14]. However, LLINs were expected to be delivered in different approaches other than bed nets considering the diurnal activity patterns of *Aedes* mosquitoes.

In Haiti, LLIN bed nets showed an immediate effect on immature-based indicators and dengue transmission and extended for the following 5–12 months after their deployment [15]. Other sets of more ample studies suggested the potential of LLIN as window curtains (insecticide-treated curtains (ITCs)) to reduce dengue vector densities to low levels and potentially impact on dengue transmission. In Thailand, ITCs showed immediate effects on immature-based indicators at 6 months [16]. Combining ITCs with targeting productive breeding sites in Mexico [17], Venezuela [17, 18] and Guatemala [19] improved the impact on *A. aegypti*. In a field trial carried out in Mexico, ITC interventions did not affect the indoor adult population, but it seemed to reduce the number of DEN-infected females and the human infection prevalence in some areas [20].

While ITCs can be easily introduced within DEN endemic areas, these studies showed, as found with bed nets, that ITCs required proper handling and use by local communities to be effective. Coverage of the interventions based on ITCs typically falls dramatically over time [16, 21, 22], undoubtedly compromising efficacy throughout the community. For example, in Iquitos, Peru, a sociological study found that proper use of ITC falls dramatically over time (45% in the second year of deploying) [21, 22]. Particularly, at the household level, the efficacy of ITCs is compromised when curtains remain open/tied back during daytime or when all house entry points cannot be protected [16–20, 23]. In Guatemala [19] and Mexico [20], it was noted that families would remove or tie back the curtains to increase ventilation during the day, compromising the utility of the intervention as *A. aegypti* is a day-biting mosquito. A solution to this is to permanently fix the LLIN to the doors and windows in the form of a screen rather than curtains [24, 25].

3. House screening

Here, we use the term house screening to refer the use of insect screens in a house. An insect screen is basically a mesh (metal wire, fibreglass or other synthetic fibres) stretched in a frame (wood or metal) fixed on the opening of a house such as a door or a window. 'Mosquito-proofing' of houses (with insect screens) is a form of environmental management based on changes to human habitation to exclude vectors and reduce man-vector-pathogen contact including mosquitoes [26, 27].

The first published work evaluating house screening as physical method to prevent mosquito-borne diseases was reported by Celli in Italy for the control of malaria among railroad workers and their families [28]. His study showed that screening porches and chimneys resulted in significant reductions on malaria incidence (4% with screens vs. 92% without the intervention) [29].

The Italian experience led to widespread screening of houses against mosquitoes in malarious areas, not only in Italy but also around the world. Examples of house screening as a malaria control intervention include workers building the Panama Canal and rural homes in the Southern United States [30]. Nevertheless, this protective and efficacious method was largely forgotten when the primary strategy of insecticidal control with DDT (dichloro-diphenyl-trichloroethane) emerged [30]. Modern studies on house screening have proven significant reductions on malaria [31–33] and described to be widely accepted by communities [34].

The integration of house screening for the control of dengue was evaluated in Vietnam in the 1990s. Nguyen et al. [35] and Igarashi [36] evaluated an intervention with permethrin nets covering all openings of houses (in addition to routine anti-*Aedes* health education and control measures) and reported a significant reduction (close to 100%) in the number of houses positive for dengue vectors. Furthermore, indoor *A. aegypti* was undetectable levels for 7 months, while in the control group, infestation gradually increased during the epidemic season, and a positive impact in preventing DEN transmission during the epidemic season (at 6 months after intervention) was observed. Therefore, screening doors and windows have been considered with the potential to limit transmission in the most recent systematic reviews [4, 9].

4. *Aedes aegypti*-proof houses

The intervention called *Aedes aegypti*-proof houses ('Casas a prueba de *Aedes aegypti*') involves insecticide-treated screening (ITS) with the use of long-lasting insecticidal nets (LLINs) permanently fitted to windows and doors to exclude *A. aegypti*, vector of dengue, chikungunya and Zika (**Figure 1**).

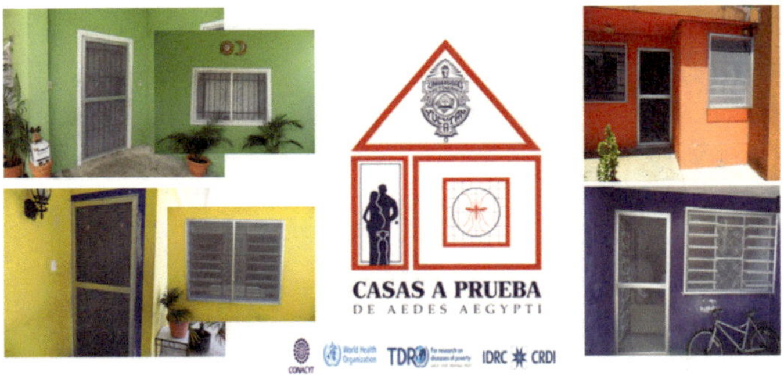

Figure 1. Photographs show *Aedes aegypti*-proof houses with insecticide-treated screens mounted on aluminium frames and fixed to external doors and windows of treated houses.

As described by Manrique-Saide et al. [24] and Che-Mendoza et al. [25], Duranet® screens (0.55% w.w. alpha-cypermethrin-treated non-flammable polyethylene netting [145 denier; mesh1⁄4132 holes/sq. inch]; Clarke Mosquito Control, Roselle, IL, USA; WHOPES approved for LLIN use) were mounted in aluminium frames custom-fitted to doors and windows of

http://dx.doi.org/10.5772/67934

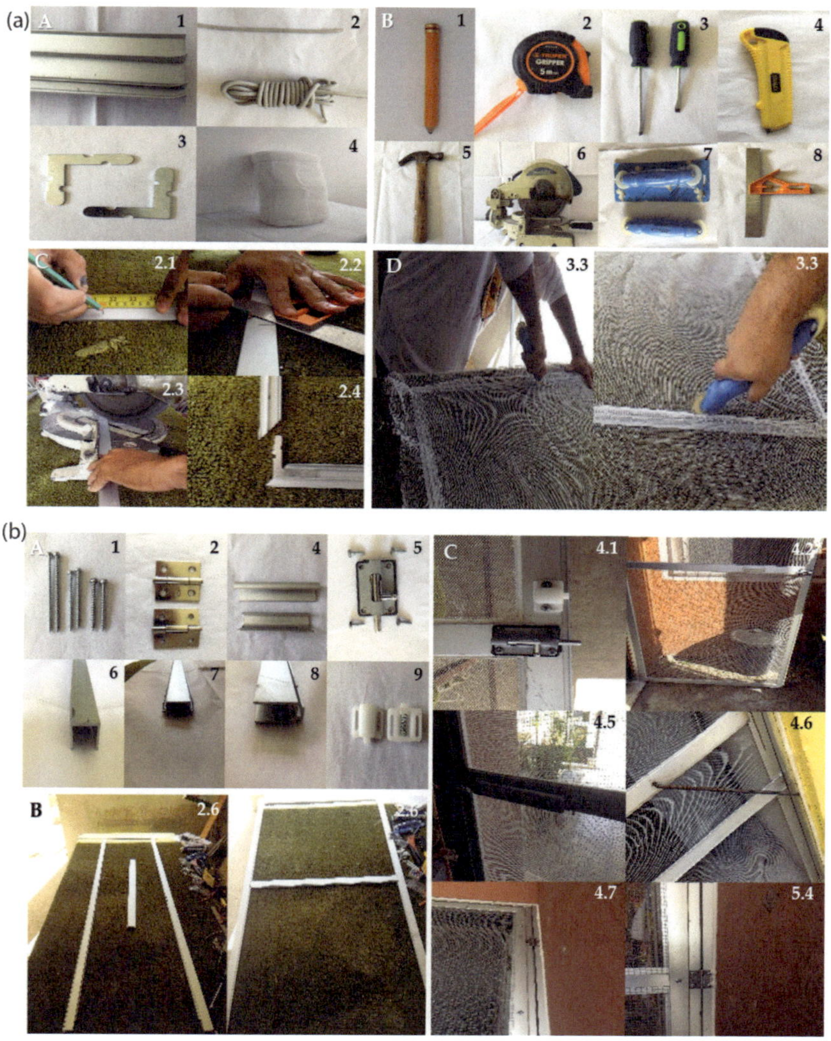

Figure 2. General description of how to install insecticide-treated screens on windows and doors. **Window: (A)** Materials required: (**1**) screen frame, (**2**) square for screen frame, (**3**) vinyl #12 and (**4**) window screen. **(B)** Tools required: (**1**) pencil, (**2**) measuring tape, (**3**) screwdriver, (**4**) sharp knife, (**5**) hammer, (**6**) hacksaw, (**7**) convex wheel and (**8**) universal square. **(C)** Step 2: (**2.1**) Using a measuring tape and pencil, make a mark where a cut is to be made on the new frame. (**2.2**) With the universal square, mark a 45° angle on the first mark of the final measure. (**2.3**) Use the hacksaw to make the 45° cut. Make four cuts, one on each side of the window. (**2.4**) Use squares to join the four parts of the frame. Insert squares into the frame along the side with 45° cut and lightly tap the squares into place. Check the assembled frame for squareness. **(D)** Step 3: (**3.3**) With the help of the convex wheel, insert the screen into the channel with vinyl, beginning at one corner (press down and roll with short strokes back and forth). When all sides have been inserted into the vinyl, remove the excess vinyl. **Door: (A)** Materials required: (**1**) screws (1 ½ × 8″, ½ × 8, 1 × 8), (**2**) hinges, (**3**) vinyl # 12, (**4**) elephant trunk handle, (**5**) hasp, (**6**) chair butt, (**7**) mosquito door frame central, (**8**) mosquito door frame vertical and (**9**) lock. **(B)** Step 2: (**2.6**) Forming the door, 1 ½ × 8 screws should preferably be used. Step 4: (**4.1**) The lock and pin are installed in the central part of the frame, at the appropriate distance for its correct operation. (**4.2**) The elephant trunk handle is installed in the central part of the frame. (**4.5**) Spring allows the automatic closing of the door. (**4.6**) Pivot allows the automatic closing of the door in a slow and controlled way. (**4.7**) Metal mesh protects the mosquito net from damage caused by animals. Step 5: (**5.4**) Fix the door to the frame using ½ × 8 screws, a drill and a screwdriver. Check the assembled door for squareness.

houses in collaboration with a local small business (**Figure 2**). An average of two doors and five windows by house were installed in each intervention cluster. During the installation, at least one person in every household received information from research staff about the proper use and maintenance of ITS.

5. Studies with ITS and protection against *A. aegypti* mosquitoes in Mexico

From 2009 to 2014, cluster randomised controlled trials were conducted in two Mexican cities—Acapulco (Guerrero state) and Merida (Yucatan state)—to test the efficacy of the intervention *Aedes aegypti*-proof houses. The first study in Acapulco was followed by a subsequent phase of scaling-up to replication in Merida as a 'horizontal' scaling-up to expand the availability of the intervention geographically.

In general, the studies compared 10 control and 10 intervention areas of 100 households each across both cities. Routine vector control activities—as implemented by the local Ministry of Health—were performed in control clusters. Intervention clusters included insecticide-treated window and door screens (Acapulco and Merida) and targeted interventions in the productive water container types (in Acapulco only). As part of the national policy in response to dengue outbreaks and entomological risk indices [37], control and ITS intervention clusters could receive routine vector control activities (outdoor spraying with the organophosphates malathion or chlorpyrifos, indoor space spraying with the pyrethroid deltamethrin or the carbamates propoxur or bendiocarb and larviciding with the organophosphate temephos).

The main outcome metrics were the reduction of indoor vector densities. Five cross-sectional entomological surveys were conducted in intervention and control clusters as in Manrique-Saide et al. [24] and Che-Mendoza et al. [25]. Briefly, indoor adult mosquito collections were performed in a randomly selected subsample of 30 houses from each cluster (total of 300 houses per arm). A baseline survey was performed prior to the installation of ITS and was followed by surveys at 6 months of intervals corresponding to dry (low vector abundance, 6 and 18 months of post-intervention (PI)) and wet (high vector abundance, 12 and 24 of months PI) seasons. Indoor adult mosquitoes were collected with Prokopack aspirators [38] for a 15-min period per house. Collections within each cluster were performed on the same day between 09:00 and 15:00 h by skilled collector teams.

The indoor *A. aegypti* adult-based entomological indicators monitored for 2 years in both localities are shown in **Figure 3**. During the pre-intervention survey, similar infestation levels were quantified in both study arms. ITS protected houses against *A. aegypti* mosquitoes: significant reduction of indoor-resting adults by approximately 50% on the presence ($OR \leq 0.62$, $P < 0.05$) and abundance ($IRR \leq 0.58$, $P < 0.05$). The combination of ITS and interventions targeting productive container types was successful in continuing reducing the number of *Aedes* pupae and consequently of adult dengue vectors.

http://dx.doi.org/10.5772/67934

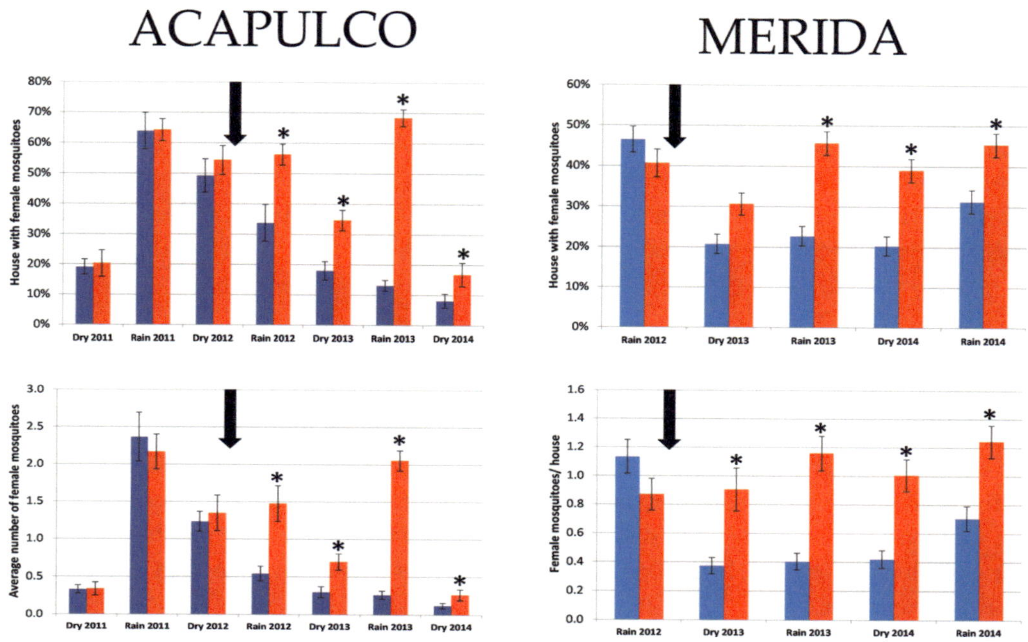

Figure 3. Comparison between groups of houses protected with insecticidetreated (blue bars) and untreated (red bars) screens on the percentage of infested houses (top) and infestation density (bottom) for female *Aedes aegypti* in Acapulco and Merida, Mexico. The blue arrow represents the start of the interventions. The symbol (*) denotes dates when the index was significantly different between treated and control groups on that date. Error bars show the standard error of the mean.

A significant effect on indoor adult *Aedes* infestations was observed in houses protected with ITS but not in controls, despite the fact that *Aedes* populations at both sites were resistant to pyrethroids, and this protection was sustained beyond 24 months when ITS was combined with targeted treatment of productive breeding sites (as demonstrated in Acapulco, where the combined intervention maintained a statistically significant protective effect on *Aedes* adult and immature stages until the end of the study, approximately 600 days after ITS installation).

Multiple factors could explain the lack of complete suppression of *A. aegypti* indoors by ITS. First, this method did not aim to reduce peridomestic breeding or abundance of mosquitoes. As intervention coverage on each block was not 100%, there is a possibility for mosquito breeding and human feeding even in the presence of screens. In Acapulco, Mexico, combining ITS with peridomestic larval control on the most productive larval breeding habitats produced a synergistic effect evidenced as a reduction of the abundance of indoor female mosquitoes in screened houses [25]. This finding provides evidence of the importance of integrating ITS with methods focused on peridomestic control. Another factor explaining indoor presence of *A. aegypti* in screened houses is the fact that maybe some adults did not contact and/or survive after the initial contact with the LLIS or probably not all contacted the screened surfaces on the day when collections were performed.

Another explanation could be the loss of insecticidal power and high pyrethroid resistance in the mosquito populations of Merida. Exposure to sunlight, rain and dust impacts the residual power of pyrethroid insecticides. Despite of this, we demonstrated in this study that insecticidal activity of ITS under operational conditions is still acceptable after 2 years of use.

The physiological resistance in mosquitoes to the insecticide and the effect on the performance of a LLIN cannot be discounted. Pyrethroid resistance in *A. aegypti* populations of Mexico, including Merida, has increased during the last decade [39–42]. Currently, ITS with LLIN will have to challenge insecticide resistance to pyrethroids because they are the only insecticide class recommended and available for LLIN [43].

6. Social acceptance and cultural barriers on *Aedes aegypti*-proof houses

In Acapulco, the social studies aimed to explore the acceptance, use, adherence and perspectives of the ITS and suggestions about how to modify the programme to better address the sociocultural needs of the community. Part of the results was published by Jones et al. [44]. The main reason for acceptance was that the screens were perceived to be beneficial. The fear of violence, particularly important in Acapulco, was frequently identified as a common reason for rejection.

The most noted benefit reported for the use of ITS in Acapulco was the reduction on the amount of mosquitoes in the houses. Following screen installation, 79.9% of recipients reported that there were fewer mosquitoes inside, and a further 10.8% reported that there were none. The reduction in the amount of indoor mosquitoes was associated with a reduction in mosquito biting: 88.5% or recipients reported that mosquito biting was less of a nuisance within their homes after receiving the screens.

Participants also appreciated a reduction in mosquito numbers. Though many were unaware that the net contained insecticide, they had noticed that mosquitoes and other pests died on contact with the screen and were satisfied with this. The insecticide in the screen was seen as beneficial and acceptable, with few reports of side effects or fears about its use. Participants reported a reduction in flies and cockroaches, and 79.9% of satisfaction survey participants reported a reduction in other pests. The majority of participants (90.2%) had the same amount or more screens in place now compared to the original amount installed, suggesting that very few were removed.

The main problem identified with the screens once installed was fragility, especially on doors. The satisfaction survey found that the most common reason for a house to have fewer screens now than originally installed was screen breakage (44%) and higher quality material was the most frequently suggested improvement for the project. A survey of the screens found that the windows were broadly in very good condition, whereas the doors were faring less well, with 42.4% damaged in some way. Some screens were broken in exceptional accidents, but the majority of breakages reported occurred during normal use. Though some participants had feared a reduction in air circulation prior to installation, none had experienced this problem. Indeed, many expressed surprise that they had felt no effect.

Overall satisfaction with the project was very high. About 80.9% scored their satisfaction with the screens as 5/5, 89.9% gave a score of 4 or 5 and 99.3% recommend the project to another city.

In Merida, we conducted an ethnographic research in a small neighbourhood called Manzana 115, where 140 households are accepted to participate in the *Aedes aegypti*-proof houses project. In addition to an acceptance or rejection study, we also investigated 'the process of decision'. The social perception on ITS efficacy was documented since the invitation to the families. Overall, 80% of families accepted the intervention in the first invitation, whereas 30% rejected it, and at least 20% decided to accept before some family consultation. The most common reasons for acceptance were (a) that the screens were perceived to be beneficial, (b) free of cost and no future charges, (c) expectation of future 'support' and (d) high-risk perception about dengue. In Merida, the most important reasons for reluctance and rejection were (a) no interest at all; (b) low perception about dengue risk infection and (c) wives did not accept the intervention because their husbands didn't authorise it. Therefore, it is important to consider the gender roles on the decision-making processes, suggesting that both men and women must be included on social understanding about innovations for family health care.

Afterwards the installation of ITS, 80% of households reported to be very satisfied and considered the intervention effective on reducing and killing mosquitoes, not toxic for humans and pets, and also considered it important because there was no temperature increase in their houses.

7. Conclusions

In the absence of effective treatment or vaccines and in the context of multiple co-circulating viruses transmitted by *Aedes* mosquitoes, the development of preventive and long-lasting methods for *Aedes* control has become a top global health priority.

The benefits of house screening, as a physical barrier, rely on its efficacy to exclude mosquitoes and eventually protect against mosquito bites, which is epidemiologically relevant if most transmission occurs indoors. From an environmental health perspective, residential premises (house and peridomicile) offer important habitats for supporting populations of *A. aegypti* as they emerge from productive breeding sites, move in and out houses in search of food (human blood), refuge and mating and oviposit at the suitable breeding sites to complete their life cycle. *Aedes* is an anthropophilic, endophilic and endophagic species, and the house is the epidemiologically most significant point of vector-human contact for arbovirus transmission.

The adaptation of long-lasting insecticide nets permanently fitted as mosquito screens on windows and doors has advantages over other approaches (such as bed nets and curtains) because these interventions are in place permanently and require little additional work or behavioural change by householders.

Our studies in Mexico demonstrate that LLIS deployed as ITS acts as a barrier and significantly restrains the entrance of mosquitoes to houses for at least 2 years post deployment. Concisely, a house protected with ITS on doors and windows has at least 50% less chances of having *A. aegypti* females in comparison with a non-protected house. ITS confirmed a sustained protective effect on indoor female mosquitoes, the most epidemiologically important target for vector control, even in the presence of high levels of resistance to pyrethroids in the local mosquito population.

The present studies provide valuable and unique information on the use of house screening within cities endemic for mosquito-borne diseases, and at the time of writing, are unique in supporting the feasibility and potential benefit of this method for the simultaneous prevention and control of dengue, chikungunya and Zika transmission. The positive results from trials using house screening/full screening of windows/doors suggest that excluding the vector *A. aegypti* from the home may prove to be an innovative approach in terms of environmental management (changes to human habitation), if it is proven ultimately to reduce transmission of the pathogens to humans. This simple classic method of vector control should be considered and encouraged by the National Ministries of Health.

As most human-mosquito contacts occur indoors, the observed reductions in abundance and prevalence of infestation in our studies may be significant enough to impact virus transmission in a measurable way. Assessing the epidemiological impact of existing and new paradigms on *Aedes*-borne disease transmission remains a top research and public health priority. Particularly for ITS, our entomological studies provide evidence for the development of robust RCT (Randomized Controlled Trials) evaluating the short- and long-term protective efficacy of this method. Of particular interest is the evaluation of the potential for ITS to be included within an IVM (Integrated Vector Management) scheme that also includes other modes of vector control that target peridomestic breeding or adult abundance (e.g. larviciding, ULV).

The authorities of Mexico are considering how to expand *Aedes aegypti*-proof housing to as many homes as possible, probably as a targeted intervention for high-risk areas (hot spots) of endemic localities. Given that the same mosquito transmits dengue, chikungunya and Zika, the local government of Yucatan is planning to scale this intervention to protect the most vulnerable, particularly pregnant women and their families. Therefore, and in accordance with the local MoH, our team is currently also developing a pilot study evaluating an integrated intervention on pregnant women, providing them with information and a kit of tools including repellents and *Aedes aegypti*-proof houses to protect them against mosquito biting and disease transmission.

Ultimately, ITS is a housing improvement that should be part of the current paradigms for urban vector-borne disease control [45].

Acknowledgements

The studies were funded by the Consejo Nacional de Ciencia y Tecnologia (Project Salud-2010-01-161551), Fondo Sectorial de Investigación en Salud y Seguridad Social (SSA/IMSS/ISSSTE-CONACYT Mexico), Fomix CONACYT-Guerrero (Project GUE-2008-02-108686), the Special Programme for Research and Training in Tropical Diseases (TDR) at the World Health Organization and the International Development Research Centre (IDRC) of Canada within the programme 'Towards Improved Dengue and Chagas Disease Control through Innovative Ecosystem Management and Community-Directed Interventions: An Eco-Bio-Social Research Programme on Dengue and Chagas Disease in Latin America and the Caribbean' (Project Number 104951–001). The nets employed in this study were donated by the company Public Health Supply and Equipment de Mexico, S.A. de C.V. Thanks to Suzanna Shugert for grammatical revision.

Author details

Pablo Manrique-Saide[1]*, Azael Che-Mendoza[1], Josué Herrera-Bojórquez[1], Josué Villegas Chim[1], Guillermo Guillermo-May[1], Anuar Medina-Barreiro[1], Felipe Dzul-Manzanilla[1], Abdiel Martín-Park[1,2], Gabriela González-Olvera[1], Hugo Delfín-Gonzalez[1], Juan I. Arredondo-Jiménez[3], Adriana E. Flores-Suarez[3], Norma Pavía-Ruz[1], Catrin Huws Jones[4], Audrey Lenhart[4] and Gonzalo Vazquez-Prokopec[5,6]

*Address all correspondence to: msaide@correo.uady.mx

1 Autonomous University of Yucatan, Merida, Yucatan, Mexico

2 Catedras-CONACYT, Autonomous University of Yucatan, Merida, Yucatan, Mexico

3 Autonomous University of Nuevo Leon, San Nicolas de los Garza, N.L., Mexico

4 Liverpool School of Tropical Medicine, Liverpool, UK

5 Centers for Disease Control and Prevention, Atlanta, GA, USA

6 Emory University, Atlanta, GA, USA

References

[1] Bosio CF, Fulton RE, Salasek ML, Beaty BJ, Black WC. Quantitative trait loci that control vector competence for dengue-2 virus in the mosquito *Aedes aegypti*. Genetics. 2000; **156**: 687-698

[2] Bhatt S, Gething PW, Brady OJ, Messina JP, Farlow AW, Moyes CL, Drake JM, Brownstein JS, Hoen AG, Sankoh O, Myers MF, George DB, Jaenisch T, Wint GR, Simmons CP, Scott TW, Farrar JJ, Hay SI. The global distribution and burden of dengue. Nature. 2013; **496**: 504-507. DOI: 10.1038/nature12060

[3] Li MI, Wong PS, Ng LC, Tan CH. Oral susceptibility of Singapore *Aedes* (*Stegomyia*) *aegypti* (Linnaeus) to Zika virus. PLoS Neglected Tropical Diseases. 2012; **6**(8): e1792. DOI: 10.1371/journal.pntd.0001792. pmid: 22953014

[4] Bowman LR, Donegan S, McCall PJ. Is Dengue Vector Control Deficient in Effectiveness or Evidence?: Systematic Review and Meta-analysis. PLoS Neglected Tropical Diseases. 2016; **10**(3): e0004551. DOI: 10.1371/journal.pntd.0004551

[5] Morrison A, Zielinski-Gutierrez E, Scott T, Rosenberg R. Defining challenges and proposing solutions for control of the virus vector *Aedes aegypti*. PLoS Medicine. 2008; **5**(3): e68. DOI: 10.1371/journal.pmed.0050068

[6] Achee NL, Gould F, Perkins TA, Reiner RC, Jr., Morrison AC, Ritchie SA, Gubler DJ, Teyssou R, Scott TW. A critical assessment of vector control for dengue prevention. PLoS Neglected Tropical Diseases. 2015; **9**: e0003655. DOI: 10.1371/journal.pmed.0050068

[7] World Health Organization. Guidelines for Laboratory and Field Testing of Long-Lasting Insecticidal Nets. Geneva: WHO. 2013; WHO/HTM/NTD/WHOPES/2013.1

[8] Lengeler C. Insecticide-treated bed nets and curtains for preventing malaria. Cochrane Database of Systematic Reviews. 2004; 2(2): 1-54. Art. No.: CD000363. DOI: 10.1002/14651858. CD000363.pub2

[9] Wilson AL, Dhiman RC, Kitron U, Scott TW, van den Berg H, Lindsay SW. Benefit of insecticide-treated nets, curtains and screening on vector borne diseases, excluding malaria: a systematic review and meta-analysis. PLoS Neglected Tropical Diseases. 2014; **8**(10): e3228. DOI: 10.1371/journal.pntd.0003228

[10] Takken W. Do insecticide-treated bednets have an effect on malaria vectors? Tropical Medicine and International Health. 2002; **7**(12): 1022-1030. DOI: 10.1046/j.1365-3156. 2002.00983.x

[11] Vanlerberghe V, Villegas E, Oviedo M, Baly A, Lenhart A, McCall PJ, Van der Stuyft P. Evaluation of the effectiveness of insecticide treated materials for household level dengue vector control. PLoS Neglected Tropical Diseases. 2011a; **5**(3): e994. DOI: 10.1371/ journal.pntd.0000994

[12] World Health Organization. Malaria Control Today: Current WHO Recommendations. Working document Roll Back Malaria Department. 2005a. Geneva: WHO. 75 p.

[13] World Health Organization. Insecticidetreated mosquito nets: a WHO position statement. [Internet]. 2005. Available from: http://www.who.int/malaria/publications/atoz/ itnspospaperfinal.pdf. [Accessed 2016/12/07]

[14] McCall PJ, Kittayapong P. Control of Dengue Vectors: Tools and Strategies. Report of the Scientific Working Group on Dengue. 2006. World Health Organization on behalf of the Special Programme for Research and Training in Tropical Diseases. [Internet]. 2007. pp. 110-119. Available from: http://www.who.int/tdr/publications/documents/swg_dengue_ 2.pdf. [Accessed 2016/10/21]

[15] Lenhart A, Orelus N, Maskill R, Alexander N, Streit T, McCall PJ. Insecticide-treated bednets to control dengue vectors: preliminary evidence from a controlled trial in Haiti. Tropical Medicine & International Health. 2008; **13**(1): 56-67. DOI: 10.1111/j.1365-3156. 2007.01966.x

[16] Vanlerberghe V, Trongtokit Y, Jirarojwatana S, Jirarojwatana R, Lenhart A, Apiwathnasorn C, McCall PJ, Van der Stuyft P. Coverage-dependent effect of insecticide-treated curtains for dengue control in Thailand. The American Journal of Tropical Medicine and Hygiene. 2013; **89**(1): 93-98. DOI: 10.4269/ajtmh.13-0015

[17] Kroeger A, Lenhart A, Ochoa M, Villegas E, Levy M, Alexander N. Effective control of dengue vectors with curtains and water container covers treated with insecticide in Mexico and Venezuela: cluster randomised trials. BMJ. 2006; **332**: 1247-1252. DOI: http:// dx.doi.org/10.1136/bmj.332.7552.1247

[18] Vanlerberghe V, Villegas E, Jirarojwatana S, Santana N, Trongtorkit Y, Jirarojwatana R, Srisupap W, Lefèvre P, Van der Stuyft P. Determinants of uptake, short term and continued use of insecticide-treated curtains and jar covers for dengue control. The American Journal of Tropical Medicine and Hygiene. 2011b; **16**: 162-173. DOI: 10.1111/j.1365-3156.2010.02668.x

[19] Rizzo N, Gramajo R, Cabrera-Escobar M, Arana B, Kroeger A, Manrique-Saide P, Petzold M. Dengue vector management using insecticide treated materials and targeted interventions on productive breeding-sites in Guatemala. BMC Public Health. 2012; **12**: 931-948. DOI: 10.1186/1471-2458-12-931

[20] Loroño-Pino MA, García-Rejón JE, Machain-Williams C, Gomez-Carro S, Nuñez-Ayala G, Nájera-Vázquez Mdel R, Losoya A, Aguilar L, Saavedra-Rodriguez K, Lozano-Fuentes S, Beaty MK, Black WC 4th, Keefe TJ, Eisen L, Beaty BJ. Towards a Casa Segura: a consumer product study of the effect of insecticide-treated curtains on *Aedes aegypti* and dengue virus infections in the home. The American Journal of Tropical Medicine and Hygiene. 2013; **89**: 385-397. DOI: 10.4269/ajtmh.12-0772

[21] Paz-Soldan VA, Bauer KM, Lenhart A, Cordova Lopez JJ, Elder JP, Scott T, McCall PJ, Kochel TJ, Morrison AC. Experiences with insecticide-treated curtains: a qualitative study in Iquitos, Peru. BMC Public Health. 2016a; **16**: 582. DOI: 10.1186/s12889-016-3191-x

[22] Paz-Soldan VA, Bauer K, Morrison AC, Cordova Lopez JJ, Izumi K, Scott TW, Elder JP, Alexander N, Halsey ES, McCall PJ, Lenhart A. Factors associated with correct and consistent insecticide treated curtain use in Iquitos, Peru. PLoS Neglected Tropical Diseases. 2016b; **10**(3): e0004409. DOI: 10.1371/journal.pntd.0004409

[23] Lenhart A, Trongtokit Y, Alexander N, Apiwathnasorn C, Satimai W, Vanlerberghe V, Van der Stuyft P, McCall PJ. A cluster-randomized trial of insecticide-treated curtains for dengue vector control in Thailand. The American Journal of Tropical Medicine and Hygiene. 2013; **88**: 254-259. DOI: 10.4269/ajtmh.2012.12-0423

[24] Manrique-Saide P, Che-Mendoza A, Barrera-Pérez M, Guillermo-May G, Herrera-Bojórquez J, Dzul-Manzanilla F, Gutierrez-Castro C, Lenhart A, Vazquez-Prokopek G, Sommerfeld J, McCall PJ, Kroeger A, Arredondo-Jiménez JI. Long-lasting insecticide treated house screens reduce domestic infestations of dengue vectors in Mexico. Emerging Infectious Diseases. 2015; **21**: 308-311. DOI: 10.3201/eid2102.140533

[25] Che-Mendoza A, Guillermo-May G, Herrera-Bojórquez J, Barrera-Pérez M, Dzul-Manzanilla F, Gutierrez-Castroc C, Arredondo-Jiménez JI, Sánchez-Tejeda G, Vazquez-Prokopec G, Ranson H, Lenhart H, Sommerfeld J, McCall PJ, Kroeger A, Manrique-Saide P. Long-lasting insecticide treated house screens and targeted treatment of productive breeding sites for dengue vector control in Acapulco, Mexico. Transactions of the Royal Society of Tropical Medicine and Hygiene. 2015; **109**: 106-115. DOI: 10.1093/trstmh/tru189

[26] World Health Organization. Manual on environmental management for mosquito control, with special emphasis on malaria vectors. 1982. WHO Offset Publication, vol. 66. Geneva

[27] Schofield CJ, Briceno-Leon R, Kolstrup N, Webb DJT, White GB. The role of house design in limiting vector-borne disease. In: Curtis CE editor. Appropriate Technology in Vector Control. CRC Press; 1990. 233 p.

[28] Celli A. La nuova profilassi della malaria nel Lazio [The new prophylaxis against malaria in Lazio]. Supplemento al Policlinico. 1900; **6**: 1601-1606

[29] Ferroni E, Jefferson T, Gachelin G. Angelo Celli and research on the prevention of malaria in Italy a century ago. Journal of the Royal Society of Medicine. 2012; **105**: 35-40. DOI: 10.1258/jrsm.2011.11k049

[30] Lindsay SW, Emerson PM, Charlwood JD. Reducing malaria by mosquito-proofing houses. Trends in Parasitology. 2002; **18**: 510-514. DOI: http://dx.doi.org/10.1016/S1471-4922(02)02382-6

[31] Kirby M, Green C, Milligan P, Sismanidis C, Jasseh M, Conway D, Lindsay S. Risk factors for house-entry by malaria vectors in a rural town and satellite villages in The Gambia. Malaria Journal. 2008; **7**: 2. DOI: 10.1186/1475-2875-7-2

[32] Kirby MJ, Ameh D, Bottomley C, Green C, Jawara M, Milligan PJ, Snell PC, Conway DJ, Lindsay SW. Effect of two different house screening interventions on exposure to malaria vectors and on anaemia in children in The Gambia: a randomised controlled trial. Lancet. 2009; **374**: 998-1009. DOI: 10.1016/S0140-6736(09)60871-0

[33] Lindsay SW, Jawara M, Paine K, Pinder M, Walraven G, Emerson PM. Changes in house design reduce exposure to malaria mosquitoes. Tropical Medicine & International Health. 2003; **8**: 512-517. DOI: 10.1046/j.1365-3156.2003.01059.x

[34] Kirby MJ, Bah P, Jones CO, Kelly AH, Jasseh M, Lindsay SW. Social acceptability and durability of two different house screening interventions against exposure to malaria vectors, *Plasmodium falciparum* infection, and anemia in children in the Gambia, West Africa. The American Journal of Tropical Medicine and Hygiene. 2010; **83**: 965-972. DOI: 10.4269/ajtmh.2010.10-0311

[35] Nguyen HT, Tien TV, Tien NC, Ninh TU, Hoa NT. The effect of Olyset net screen to control the vector of dengue fever in Vietnam. Dengue Bulletin. 1996; **20**: 87-92.

[36] Igarashi A. Impact of dengue virus infection and its control. FEMS Immunology & Medical Microbiology. 1997; **18**: 291-300. DOI: http://dx.doi.org/10.1111/j.1574-695X.1997.tb01058.x

[37] Hernández-Ávila JE, Rodrıíguez M-H, Santos-Luna R, Sánchez-Castañeda V, Román-Pérez S, Ríos-Salgado VH, Salas-Sarmiento JA. Nation-wide, web-based, geographic information system for the integrated surveillance and control of dengue fever in Mexico. PLOS One. 2013; **8**(8): e70231. DOI: 10.1371/annotation/fa2d8273-9377-44c0-b61f-eb019beca2ce

[38] Vazquez-Prokopec GM, Galvin WA, Kelly R, Kitron U. A new, cost-effective, battery-powered aspirator for adult mosquito collections. Journal of Medical Entomology. 2009; **46**: 1256-1259. DOI: http://dx.doi.org/10.1603/033.046.0602

[39] González G, Ponce G, Quiroz-Martínez H, García JE, Flores AE. Insecticide resistance mechanisms in *Aedes aegypti* from Merida, Yucatan, Mexico, related with two dengue transmission seasons. Journal of American Mosquito Control Association. 2012; **28**: 103.

[40] Ponce-García GP, Flores AE, Fernández-Salas I, Saavedra-Rodríguez K, Reyes-Solis G, Lozano-Fuentes S, Guillermo Bond J, Casas-Martínez M, Ramsey JM, García-Rejón J, Domínguez-Galera M, Ranson H, Hemingway J, Eisen L, Black IV WC. Recent rapid rise of a permethrin knock down resistance allele in *Aedes aegypti* in México. PLoS Neglected Tropical Diseases. 2009; **3**(10): e531. DOI: 10.1371/journal.pntd.0000531

[41] Saavedra-Rodríguez K, Beaty M, Lozano-Fuentes S, Denham S, Garcia-Rejon J, Reyes-Solis G, Machain-Williams C, Loroño-Pino MA, Flores-Suarez A, Ponce-Garcia G, Beaty B, Eisen L, Black IV WC. Local evolution of pyrethroid resistance offsets gene flow among *Aedes aegypti* collections in Yucatan State, Mexico. The American Society of Tropical Medicine and Hygiene. 2014; **92**: 201-209. DOI: 10.4269/ajtmh.14-0277

[42] Flores-Suarez A, Ponce-Garcia G, Lopez-Monroy B, Villanueva-Segura O, RodriguezSanchez P, Arredondo-Jimenez JI, Manrique-Saide P. Current status of the insecticide resistance in *Aedes aegypti* (Diptera: Culicidae) from Mexico. In: Trdan S editor. Insecticides Resistance. InTech Editors; 2016. pp. 99-109. Croatia, EU. DOI: 10.5772/61526

[43] Hougard JM, Duchon S, Darriet F, Zaim M, Rogier C, Guillet P. Comparative performances, under laboratory conditions, of seven pyrethroid insecticides used for impregnation of mosquito nets. Bulletin of World Health Organization. 2003; **81**: 324-333. DOI: https://dx.doi.org/10.1590/S0042-96862003000500006

[44] Jones C, Benítez-Valladares D, Barrera-Pérez M, Selem-Salas C, Chablé-Santos J, Dzul-Manzanilla F, Che-Mendoza A, Guillermo-May G, Medina-Barreiro A, Sommerfeld J, Kroeger A, Manrique-Saide P. Use and acceptance of long lasting insecticidal nets for dengue prevention in Acapulco, Guerrero, Mexico. BMC Public Health. 2014; **14**: 846. DOI: 10.1186/1471-2458-14-846

[45] Vazquez-Prokopec G, Lenhart A, Manrique-Saide P. Housing improvement: a renewed paradigm for urban vector-borne disease control? Transactions of the Royal Society of Tropical Medicine and Hygiene. 2016; **110**: 567-569. DOI: 10.1093/trstmh/trw070

Chapter 7

The Regulation Requirement of Dengue Vaccines

Yuan-Chuan Chen, Hwei-Fang Cheng,
Yi-Chen Yang and Ming-Kung Yeh

Additional information is available at the end of the chapter

http://dx.doi.org/10.5772/67744

Abstract

Dengue fever (dengue), a mosquito-borne disease caused by dengue viruses (DENVs), represents severe public health problems in Southeast Asia, Latin America, Africa and other subtropical regions. Many regulatory issues arise along with the development of dengue vaccines. It is required to follow the regulatory pathway for the license application. Dengue vaccines can be approved without local clinical phase III data. The national regulatory authorities (NRAs) must have the information, training and ability to review and approve the application. A novel vaccine product Dengvaxia® for dengue has been approved in many countries. The approval is based on clinical trials that show the vaccine could reduce about 60% dengue, prevented 90% of severe cases and 80% of hospitalizations. Several other DNA, live-attenuated, purified inactivated, subunit, vectored and chimeric vaccine candidates are currently developing in clinical phases. Although there are still some challenges for the development and regulation of vaccine, the prospects of dengue vaccines are promising provided that we can overcome the difficulty.

Keywords: dengue fever (dengue), dengue virus, dengue vaccine, clinical application

1. Introduction

In this section, we describe some background about dengue fever (dengue).

1.1. Pathogens, vectors and symptoms

Dengue, a mosquito-borne disease, is widespread all over the world in recent years. It is caused by the dengue virus (DENV), which is transmitted by female *Aedes* mosquitoes of species *A. aegypti* and *A. albopictus*. The mosquito becomes infected when it bites a person with DENVs in their blood. DENVs are maintained in cycles that involve blood-sucking vectors and vertebrate hosts. Dengue is transmitted by vectors and is not spread from one person to another person directly (**Figure 1**).

DENV, which belongs to genus *Flavivirus* of family *Flaviviridae,* is a small single-stranded RNA (ssRNA) virus comprising four distinct but closely related serotypes (DENV-1, 2, 3 and 4) [1, 2]. However, the fifth serotype DENV-5, which may be produced by genetic recombination, natural selection and genetic bottlenecks, has been discovered in 2013. This new variant follows the sylvatic cycle unlike the other four serotypes, which follow the human cycle [3].

Symptomatic DENV infections were classified into three categories: undifferentiated fever (UF), dengue fever (DF, dengue) and dengue haemorrhagic fever (DHF) (also called severe dengue). DHF was further classified into four severity grades, with grades III and IV being defined as dengue shock syndrome (DSS) [4]. Sometimes, the infection causes flu-like symptoms, which are mild, is called UF. DF begins 4–6 days after infection and its symptoms are

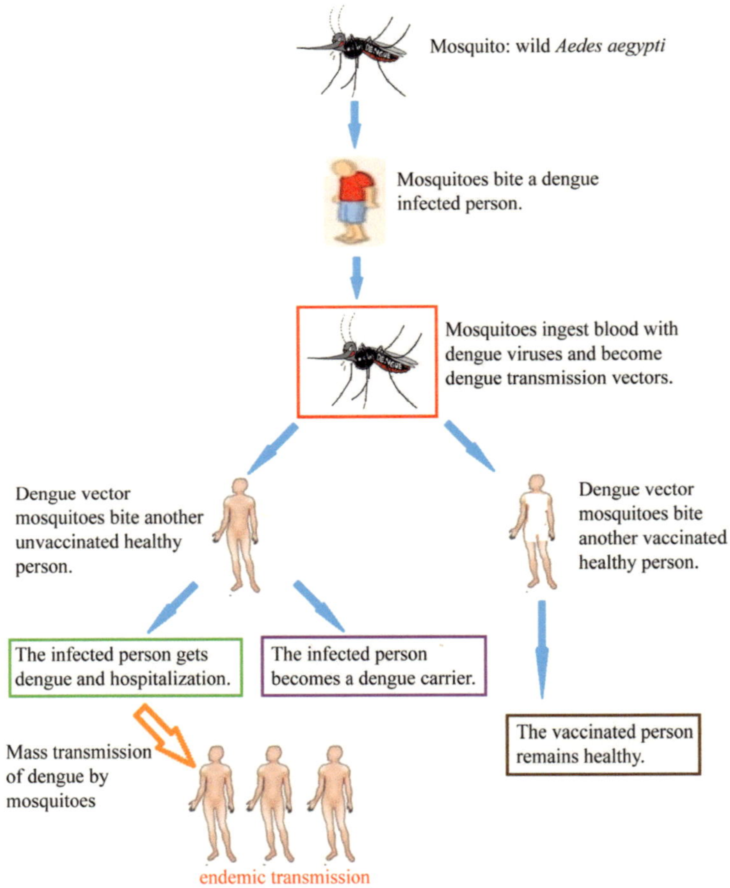

Figure 1. Dengue transmission: *Aedes* mosquitoes (*A. aegypti or A. albopictus*) bite a dengue-infected person and suck his blood. The mosquitoes ingest blood with dengue viruses and become transmission vectors after 8–10 days. The dengue vector mosquitoes bite another unvaccinated healthy person and the person gets dengue 4–13 days later. This may lead to endemic transmission if dengue is extensively spread by mosquitoes.

usually limited. However, serious problems can develop and occasionally result in a lethal complication called DHF. The symptoms may further progress to DSS, which is characterized by massive bleeding, shock and even lead to death.

Different DENV serotypes may cause a cross-serotypic immune response such as antibody-dependent enhancement (ADE). ADE is the most widely known example, which occurs in the setting of DENV infection. When an individual has been infected with one DENV serotype, the antibodies to the previous serotype will interfere with the immune responses to the new serotype to lead to more virus attack and entry. The disease varies in severity in humans from DF, which is usually limited in symptoms to lethal cases including DHF and DSS.

1.2. Epidemiology

Dengue is one of the most rapidly spreading mosquito-borne viral diseases in the world. The number of dengue cases reported annually to WHO increased from 0.4 to 1.3 million from 1996 to 2005 and reached 2.2 million and 3.2 million in 2010 and 2015, respectively [5]. The disease is currently common in more than 110 countries, mainly in Southeast Asia, Latin America, Africa, etc. Infections are usually acquired in the urbans, but they have expanded to villages, towns and cities recently.

Most people with dengue recover without any problems. The fatality rate is 1–5%, and less than 1% with adequate treatment. Because of urbanization, population growth, frequent international travelling and global warming, the incidence rate of dengue increased about 30-fold from 1960 to 2010 [6]. This disease inflicts a serious healthy, social and economic burden on the people of endemic areas.

1.3. Treatment

The treatment is only supportive and there is no certain treatment for dengue. Current efforts are to develop antiviral drugs that would be used for the treatment of dengue and prevention of severe complications. There are several plausible therapeutic approaches such as the inhibition of the viral RNA-dependent RNA polymerase inhibitor, viral protease inhibitors, entry inhibitors that stop the virus entering cells or inhibitors of the 5′ capping process, which is required for viral replication. Supportive care and adjuvant therapy may be needed in severe dengue (DHF and DSS).

1.4. Prevention and control

For dengue prevention, traditional method is only restricted to vector control measures. The best way is to inhibit the spread of the *Aedes* mosquitoes and avoid being bitten by them. This may be done by eliminating the mosquitoes, removing or covering standing water and wearing clothing that covers the body.

Integrated vector management (IVM) program is a strategy to control vectors recommended by the World Health Organization (WHO). IVM considers the following five key elements in the management process [5]:

(1) Advocacy, social mobilization and legislation: The promotion of developmental policies, the establishment or strengthening of regulatory controls for public health and the empowerment of communities.

(2) Collaboration within the health sector and with others: The consideration of all options for collaboration, strengthening communication among policy-makers, program managers and other key partners.

(3) Integrated approach to disease control: The assurance of the rational use of available resources, integration of non-chemical and chemical control methods and integration with other disease control measures.

(4) Decision based on evidence: The adaptation of strategies and interventions to local vector ecology, epidemiology and resources, guided by operational research and subject to routine monitoring and evaluation.

(5) Capacity-building: The development of essential infrastructure, adequate finance and human resources.

Vaccination is a better measure than the vector control for dengue prevention. The development of a dengue vaccine actually represents a great achievement in the control of the disease. The impact of dengue is so enormous that its vaccine development is very crucial for public health. To develop a dengue vaccine, we have to realize the regulation requirements of vaccines such as basic research, animal studies and clinical trials, etc.

2. Regulation

Dengue vaccines, as all vaccine products regulated by national regulatory authorities (NRAs) and national control laboratories (NCLs), undergo a rigorous review of laboratory and clinical data to ensure their safety, efficacy and potency. The discovery and application of dengue vaccines should follow the frame work of vaccine research and development. The manufacturer has to comply with the related regulation, including nonclinical work, preclinical trials, human clinical trials and post-market surveillance [7]. In this section, we review the regulations that are specific and required for dengue vaccines, including basic requirements, regulatory pathways, special procedures, regulatory requirement summary and regulatory challenges.

2.1. Basic requirements

The WHO Initiative for Vaccine Research (IVR) focuses on the following objectives for dengue vaccine development:

(1) Knowledge and research: Identification of knowledge gaps and research need to be related to the development, evaluation and implementation of dengue vaccines.

(2) Consensus and guidance: The scientific consensus for dengue control and guidelines on the evaluation of dengue vaccines need to be established.

(3) Review and evaluation: The evidence base for the policy recommendations related to the introduction of dengue vaccines need to be reviewed and evaluated previously.

(4) Vaccination program: The guidance and program on dengue vaccine administration, including implementation strategies need to be strictly conducted.

(5) Support of NRAs: The NRAs should be assisted and encouraged in the review of dengue vaccine registration files.

2.2. Regulatory pathways

The regulators of developing countries and developers for dengue vaccines had two meetings in 2007. The first meeting with Developing Countries' Vaccine Regulators Network (DCVRN) was held on April 2007 in Brazil [8]. Their topics included the nature and epidemiology of the dengue fever, the status of dengue vaccine development and the regulatory issues needed to be addressed. The second meeting was held in Thailand on December 2007 and several dengue vaccine developers participated in this meeting [8]. Each of these companies presented the development status of their candidates and outlined the issue that they regard important for testing and want ultimate regulatory approval of these vaccines. The summary points for their meeting report are as follows [8]:

(1) Regulatory agencies need to address some issues related to multivalent vaccines because a dengue vaccine is tetravalent and provide protection against all the four DENV serotypes.

(2) The potential risk of inducing antibody-enhanced diseases such as ADE should be verified by long-term safety assessment.

(3) Dengue vaccines need to be assessed in diverse populations because the epidemiology and impact of dengue are varied in different countries.

(4) The NRAs in developing countries may be involved in review of the applications of clinical evaluation and the marketing of vaccines and they should receive support as appropriate.

(5) Manufacturers must submit a dossier to the NRAs for review.

(6) The NRAs need to have access to the necessary expertise to review the quality and safety of dengue vaccines and consider accelerating their introduction.

(7) The improved standardized tests should be introduced for the diagnosis of early infection and for the measurement of immune protection.

On October 2009, WHO and the Pediatric Dengue Vaccine Initiative (PDVI) convened a meeting in Thailand. The topics covered in this meeting considered the interactions between scientific regulatory reviews and ethics committee reviews of applications to undertake clinical trials of dengue vaccines. Their main conclusion was that it would be better if scientific and ethical reviews can work together well, but there was no alteration in scientific or technical views about the regulation of dengue vaccines.

On October 2011, WHO convened a consultation of experts in dengue vaccine regulations to review the current scientific data regarding safety concerns associated with the live attenuated dengue vaccine. It was emphasized that a complete plan and a suitable method for long-term safety assessment are required to ensure the introduction and continuous application of dengue vaccines.

On July 2016, WHO issued a position paper to mention that countries are encouraged to establish a functional pharmacovigilance system to monitor and manage adverse reactions following immunization when dengue vaccines were introduced. Countries considering vaccination should also have a dengue surveillance system which is capable of detecting hospitalization and severe dengue cases consistently [5].

2.3. Special procedures

At the dengue vaccine development stage, some clinical trials can be omitted, although many issues regarding implementation of dengue vaccines still need to be addressed. For example, a dengue vaccine can be approved without local clinical phase III data but adopt other country's data in some countries such as Indonesia. Some vaccine candidates have progressed from animal trials directly to human clinical phase II and III in some countries such as India.

2.4. Summary of regulation requirements

It is crucial to select suitable sites for clinical trials of dengue vaccine candidates. The key consideration for selecting sites in developing countries where dengue is endemic includes investigator experience, DENV prevalence, NRA competence, the implications between rural and urban sites, acquisition of multi-year data on dengue incidence and the ability to detect clinical dengue cases. The PDVI is working with these sites in developing countries to enhance their capabilities to undertake clinical studies and safety surveillance. Many important issues have been identified for regulatory review of dengue vaccines. Plans are being developed to provide appropriate training to the NRAs to build their review capacity. Based on the results of the PDVI/DCVRN meetings on dengue vaccines, the regulation requirement of dengue vaccines is summarized as follows [8, 9]:

(1) Diligent safety surveillance: Because of possible immune enhancement in individuals who are only partially immunized and become naturally infected or who have been previously infected and receive a first vaccine dose, it is required to frequently monitor the safety of dengue vaccines in the initial stages of clinical trials. Improved definitions of adverse events following immunization are needed. In addition, methods to detect these events should be validated. It is necessary to perform improved safety surveillance and early viral analysis in cases of dengue fever.

(2) Assurance a favourable risk-benefit for the specific country: The NRAs in dengue-prevalent countries must consider new approaches to accelerate vaccine development. They will be requested to discuss on licensure of a tetravalent dengue vaccine with demonstrated efficacy and safety against only one DENV serotype. However, under this condition, post-marketing surveillance for safety and efficacy against all four serotypes is required.

http://dx.doi.org/10.5772/67744

(3) The vaccines used in testing and clinics should be the same: Vaccines being tested in subsequent studies should be the same as those being used in earlier clinical stages. Any changes in manufacturing processes or formulation are critical and could result in the need to repeat the clinical trials or require complex studies.

(4) "Standard definitions" should be commonly understood: Standardized testing methods for antibody responses and virus typing are essential, especially for laboratory-based serological tests. The validated international reference standards need to be established. In addition, phase IIa, phase IIb and phase III trials should be clearly defined.

(5) An animal model is not necessarily required: The development of an animal model would be of great benefit but likely not essential for licensure. Clinical trials could provide data to help the NRAs to understand the science of the possible severe immune-enhanced disease and identify correlates of immunity/protection that would assist vaccine development.

(6) Characteristics of clinical trial design should be defined: An effort to design clinical trial and consult the NRAs is the duty of the vaccine manufacturers. These issues include target age group for immunization, vaccine dosage schedule, trial duration and follow-up, possible immune responses to other flaviviruses, diagnosis and case definition and long-term safety surveillance. Additional considerations for assessing potential trial sites include the prevalence of the viral strains, influence of concurrent mosquito control programs, community involvement, and virological and diagnostic services.

(7) Phase III trials data can be conditionally omitted: For vaccine approval, the responsible NRAs need to establish special procedures to review and accept other country data. Phase III trials may be undertaken in some countries based on the safety and efficacy data from Phase II (a or b) trials in other countries.

(8) Joint review of license applications is recommended: The DCVRN prefers the formal procedures for collaboration and joint review of clinical trial monitoring including good clinical practice (GCP) inspections by the responsible NRAs, European Medicine Agency (EMA) and/or United States Food Drug Administration (US FDA) with facilitation by WHO. The NRAs would need to have access to the necessary expertise and advisory committee to review the quality, efficacy and safety aspects of the license application.

2.5. Regulatory challenges

The development of dengue vaccines in developing countries has been recently accelerated due to the substantial funding increase from public institutions and private sources. Along with the progress of vaccine development, two complex regulatory issues arise as follows [8]:

(1) Clinical trials data are limited in developing countries: Dengue is prevalent only in tropical countries where there is poor public health. It is almost impossible to perform clinical trials for dengue vaccines in developed countries. Clinical trials to assess the safety and efficacy of dengue vaccines are usually carried out in developing countries where dengue is prevalent, and the first licensure of dengue vaccines will occur there.

(2) Regulatory review and license approval are challenging in developing countries: It is required to ensure that developing countries have the ability to undertake appropriate regulatory review of proposed clinical studies and of applications for licensure. The NRAs of these developing countries must have the information, training and capabilities to review clinical trials and approve applications eventually.

3. Product

In this section, we introduce the newly licensed dengue vaccine in endemic countries and some developing dengue vaccines based on the regulation requirements.

3.1. Philosophy of development

Dengue has become an increasing threat around the world along with the transmission of the disease-carrying mosquitoes and the itinerary to dengue-endemic areas. To reduce the social and economic burden of dengue, before 2020, WHO aims to decrease the overall dengue mortality and morbidity by 50 and 25%, respectively. In the absence of specific antiviral therapy, effective vector control is the only strategy to mitigate the incidence rate of dengue. Vector control interventions have not been satisfied in reducing dengue transmission due to increasing rural-urban migration, rapid population growth, unplanned urbanisation and insecticide resistance in mosquitoes. The need for an effective dengue vaccine is obvious because a safe, efficacious and economic dengue vaccine can be a supplementary measure for dengue prevention and control. Vaccine development focuses on the generation of a tetravalent vaccine to provide long-term protection against the four DENV serotypes (DENV-1, 2, 3 and 4). Additionally, vaccination of target groups such as travellers and migratory population may be a suitable strategy to prevent the spread of dengue to non-endemic areas or dengue-free regions. However, there was no commercially available dengue vaccine before 2015.

3.2. Successful product: Dengvaxia®

The first dengue vaccine, known as Dengvaxia® (CYD-TDV) by Sanofi Pasteur, was registered in Mexico on December 2015 and has been licensed in many countries, including Mexico, Brazil, Philippines, El Salvador, Costa Rica, Guatemala, Peru, Indonesia, Paraguay and Singapore till 2016. It is approved for use for those aged 9–45 and recommended to prevent four DENV serotypes (DENV-1, 2, 3, and 4) [10–12].

The significant reduction in disease burden using Dengvaxia® has been demonstrated in recent research. For individuals that have been already exposed to at least one DENV, the vaccination program is most effective. Immunological screening of the population prior to vaccination is recommended. When the vaccine is given only to partial immune individuals, disease burden decreases considerably. Vaccination strategies must be planned based on epidemiological disease dynamics for each specific endemic region [10].

3.3. Production of Dengvaxia®

Dengvaxia® is designed to induce the immune system to produce antibodies against all four DENV serotypes (DENV-1, 2, 3, and 4). It is a live attenuated tetravalent chimeric vaccine developed using recombinant DNA technology by replacing the PrM (pre-membrane) and E (envelope) structural genes of the yellow fever live attenuated vaccine [10, 11]. For the vaccine, the virus is genetically engineered to include genes encoding for dengue proteins. Its production is based on a weakened combination of the yellow fever virus and each of the four DENV serotypes.

3.4. Efficacy of Dengvaxia®

Dengvaxia® was given as a three-dose series on a 0/6/12 month schedule and has been evaluated in two Phase III clinical trials. The results have been proved for each trial and pooled. The recent research has found that the vaccine was effective in reducing about 60% dengue, 65.6–81.9% hospitalization and in preventing 80–90% of DHF cases in individuals 9-45 years old [2, 10, 11].

3.5. Disadvantages of Dengvaxia®

The transmission dynamic model and clinical trial data have demonstrated that Dengvaxia® effectiveness depends mainly on the age group vaccinated and local transmission intensity [10]. Therefore, the new vaccine still has some disadvantages as follows:

(1) Reduction rate is low: In clinical trials, the vaccine only reduced the chances of developing the disease by about 60%.

(2) Not effective for all ages: The vaccine is only approved for use in people 9–45 years old. In fact, the vaccine seems to be least effective in children younger than 9 who need the vaccines most.

(3) Side effects possibly occur: Vaccinated individuals potentially have more severe cases of dengue if they contact DENVs later in life.

3.6. Developing products

Several other DNA vaccine, live-attenuated vaccine, inactivated vaccine, subunit vaccine and chimeric vaccine candidates are being developed at early stages of clinical trials by some manufacturers (**Table 1**) [13–15]. Other vaccines using virus vectors and virus-like particles (VLP) are being evaluated in preclinical studies [15].

(1) DNA vaccine: DNA vaccine candidates have been used to induce cellular immunity against various antigens using *in vitro* or animal models. This technology is based on cloning a specific gene into a bacterial plasmid containing a strong promoter for expression in mammalian cells.

(2) Live-attenuated vaccine: Live attenuated vaccine candidates, made of weakened viruses, are excellent immunogens because they can induce both humoural and cellular immune responses similar to a natural infection, but their virulence is not enough to cause diseases.

(3) Inactivated vaccine: Inactivated vaccine candidates, made from viruses inactivated by heating or formaldehyde, are safer than live-attenuated candidates because of their inability of virulence reversion and no harm to immunocompromised individuals. A synergistic formulation with another live attenuated vaccine candidate (prime-boost strategy) is being evaluated.

(4) Subunit vaccine: Recombinant subunit vaccine candidates, made of viral protein subunits, have wider safety profile. They will not produce the same immune responses as live attenuated vaccines because they contain only one or few viral proteins. The DENV envelope protein is the most immunogenic and usually used for vaccine production.

(5) Chimeric vaccine: Chimeric yellow fever/dengue virus vaccine candidates are the most advanced vaccine, being evaluated on large-scale clinical trials worldwide. These are categorised as follows:

   a. The chimeric live attenuated DENV-2/DENV vaccine (DENVax): The DENVax was constructed using the backbone of attenuated DENV-2 (PDK-53 strain) in cell culture, in which the prM and E genes of DENV-2 PDK-53 were substituted for those of wild-type DENV-1, 3 or 4.

   b. The chimeric live attenuated DENV/DENV vaccine (TetraVax-DV): The TetraVax-DV is a tetravalent vaccine candidate for which attenuation was achieved by deleting 30 nucleotides on 3′ untranslated region of wild-type DENV-1 and DENV-4. This approach did not result in any attenuation for the other two serotypes: DENV-2 and DENV-3.

(6) Vectored vaccine: The vectored vaccine candidates, a recombinant poxviruses and adenoviruses expressing foreign proteins, have been demonstrated to induce strong humoural and cellular responses in humans. Several live virus vectors such as adenovirus, alphavirus and vaccinia virus have been engineered to express DENV E protein for further evaluation as dengue vaccine candidates.

3.7. Challenges of vaccine development

Though Dengvaxia® has been successfully developed and licensed in many countries, dengue vaccine development is time-consuming, costly and difficult. The following challenges are still ahead of us for the development of new dengue vaccines [15, 16].

(1) Restriction of virus growth: The DENV is growing poorly in cell culture.

(2) Limitation in immunization: Infection by one of the four DENV serotypes will provide lasting protection against homotypic reinfection, but only transient protection against a secondary heterotypic infection.

Vaccine candidate	DEN-Vax	TetraVax-DV	TDEN PIV	V180
Type	Chimeric vaccine	Chimeric vaccine	Inactivated vaccine	Subunit vaccine
Trait	A recombinant chimeric vaccine with DENV-1, 3 and 4 components on DENV-2 backbones	A tetravalent admixture of monovalent vaccines that were tested separately for safety and immunogenicity	An inactivated tetravalent vaccine	A recombinant subunit vaccine expressed in Drosophila cells
Ongoing clinical trial	Phase I and II	Phase I and II	Phase I and II	Phase I
Testing country, company or institute	United States, Colombia, Puerto Rico, Singapore and Thailand	Thailand and Brazil	GSK and the Walter Reed Army Institute of Research	Merck

Table 1. Dengue vaccine candidates under development and on clinical trials.

(3) Incidence of antibody-enhanced diseases: The existence of four distinct DENV serotypes is capable of eliciting cross-reactive and ADE against the remaining three serotypes.

(4) Lack of an animal model: A suitable animal for dengue vaccine studies is currently not available and may result in uncertainty for the correlates of protection.

(5) Variation of the efficacy evaluation data: The neutralising antibody response to a specific DENV serotype is traditionally detected by plaque reduction neutralisation test (PRNT), but PRNT variations often occur in the collaborative studies. The variation may account for erroneous results in vaccine efficacy evaluation. Standardised guidelines need to be established by regulatory bodies like WHO for conducting PRNT.

(6) Complexity of tetravalent vaccines: Dengue is mainly caused by four DENV serotypes; thus, an effective dengue vaccine must be tetravalent. Theoretically, it is possible for inducing immune responses in individuals not protected against all four serotypes. However, the tetravalent vaccine development is difficult and complicated because of interference among the viruses.

(7) Emergency of more DENV serotypes: Discovery of DENV variants such as a sylvatic strain DENV-5 may impede the dengue vaccine initiative. Further genetic variability, ecology and epidemiology studies of these new strains are needed for the effective dengue vaccine development.

4. Perspectives

For successful vaccine introduction, it is essential to have early preparation and understanding of the true burden of dengue. Although a licensed dengue vaccine-Dengvaxia® has been available, there is need to ensure that appropriate surveillance is maintained to monitor its efficacy, safety and effectiveness during the post-licensure period. An evidence-based approach is recommended to enhance and harmonize critical characteristic of dengue vaccines including case classification, data analysis and laboratory testing. The strengthening vaccination policy will require more investment in current public health systems; furthermore, R&D, advocacy and regulation requirements of vaccines should be emphasized. The increasing knowledge and technology will provide more insights to improve vaccine design and quality. If the following prospective comes true, the effect and impact of dengue vaccines will be significant.

4.1. Enhancement of efficacy and safety

Vaccine efficacy against dengue seemed to vary according to the serotype of the infecting DENV [17]. Additional pooled efficacy, integrated safety analyses from the clinical phase III efficacy studies and the ongoing safety studies should be used to confirm the efficacy and longer term safety of dengue vaccines.

4.2. Enlargement of preventive age range

In recent studies, age-related patterns for dengue vaccine efficacy were observed in the pooled estimated efficacies against severe dengue [17]. The prevention of dengue infection caused by four DENV serotypes in individuals mainly aged 9–45 years. It would be better if the vaccine can be improved to provide significant protection to those whose age is below 9 and over 45.

4.3. Improvement of quality control

The quality control of dengue vaccines is as important as the evaluation of their efficacy. Dengue vaccines currently are not included in any pharmacopoeia. Their production, characterization, identification, test and assay should be defined in the official pharmacopoeia. Vaccine manufacturers, testing laboratories and the NRAs must strictly follow the compendial definition, methods and guidance.

4.4. Development of multivalent vaccines

If someone exposes to only one DENV serotype and specific immunity is induced to protect against this serotype, the individual protected against only one serotypes may be subjected to a severe immune response such as ADE once the individual exposes to the other serotypes. The major hindrance of dengue vaccine development is the complex immune responses to DENVs and the difficulty in eliciting concomitant protection against all distinct DENV serotypes. It would be the best to develop a multivalent vaccine against all the DENV serotypes including DENV-1, 2, 3, 4 and 5 or more, not only restricted to some serotypes.

4.5. Implementation of post-market surveillance

The dengue vaccine should be closely monitored to ensure its persistent efficacy and safety after marketing. The vaccine approved for clinical application may be required to perform additional studies to give further evaluation and often address specific questions such as safety, efficacy or possible side effects and contraindications. Local and global capacity for assessing the long-term safety of the dengue vaccine in post-licensing surveillance must be strengthened to meet the challenges imposed by its potentially complex performance [17].

4.6. Revision or enactment of related regulations

Regulatory requirements of dengue vaccine must be flexible and specific in developing countries. Continuous revision or enactment of guidelines, regulations and laws for dengue vaccines is needed to expedite new vaccine discovery. Conditional license approval should be set up and clearly defined in that the dengue transmission is diverse in different countries and local areas. In addition, the mechanisms of professional review and international cooperation for vaccine clinical application must be established.

5. Conclusions

Although many developmental and regulatory challenges are confronted, the dengue vaccine discovery is rapid and efficient. The product Dengvaxia® has been approved in several countries and a number of vaccine candidates are being developed in different phases of clinical trials. Efficacy of the vaccine candidates is variable due to varying epidemiology of the disease in diverse populations. The situation may further be complicated by the emergency of a new serotype of DENV such as DENV-5 which is different from the original four serotypes (DENV-1, 2, 3 and 4) was isolated. Sustained transmission of a new serotype may become another obstacle in the future development of dengue vaccines. Hence, it is required to strengthen the surveillance of the disease prior to any dengue vaccine is introduced into the clinical application. The safety of vaccines in clinical trials should be evaluated for longer period of time and larger populations should be involved because of its potential risk of inducing immune enhancement such as ADE. In addition, it is urgent to develop and standardise diagnostic approaches for better prediction of the protective immune responses in dengue.

Regulations are the most important criteria for the development and marketing of dengue vaccines. Regulatory science is evidence-based and any improvement or change should be dependent on scientific data. Therefore, more epidemiological and clinical data for DENV are essential for dengue vaccine research and development (R&D). Continuous revision or establishment of flexible and specific laws, regulations and guidance for dengue vaccines will expedite new vaccine discovery. Dengue is usually prevalent in developing countries with diverse social, cultural, economic and scientific development. Also, the dengue epidemiology and disease burden are quite different in these countries. Every country has specific conditions for dengue transmission, prevention and control, regulations for dengue vaccines should be enacted and implemented in accordance with the needs of individual countries and the situation of local circumstances.

In spite of some limitations, the collaborative effects of regulatory bodies such as WHO, PDVI and policy makers with vaccine manufacturers to facilitate vaccine R&D and standardize field trials are significant. The NRAs are working together to cooperate with the vaccine manufacturers to accelerate dengue vaccine development and standardise their testing. The current object is to strengthen the dengue surveillance network, explore the social and economic burden of dengue, identify clinical trial areas and support basic research to produce safe and effective dengue vaccines. In the near future, dengue vaccination may become an effectively preventive measure to substitute for vector control to suppress the increasing global burden of dengue.

Author details

Yuan-Chuan Chen[1], Hwei-Fang Cheng[1], Yi-Chen Yang[1] and Ming-Kung Yeh[2,3]*

*Address all correspondence to: mkyeh2004@gmail.com

1 Food and Drug Administration, Ministry of Health and Welfare, Taipei, Taiwan

2 School of Pharmacy, National Defense Medical Center, Taipei, Taiwan

3 Department of Public Health, Fu Jen Catholic University, New Taipei, Taiwan

References

[1] Rodenhuis-Zybert IA, Wilschut J, Smit JM. Dengue virus life cycle: viral and host factors modulating infectivity. Cellular and Molecular Life Sciences. 2010; 67(16): 2773-2786. doi: 10.1007/s00018-010-0357-z

[2] Huang SS, Li IH, Hong PD, Yeh MK. Evaluation of protective efficacy using a non-structural protein Ns1 in DNA vaccine-loaded microspheres against dengue 2 virus. International Journal of Nanomedicine. 2013; 8: 3161-3169. doi:org/10.2147/IJN.S49972

[3] Mustafa MS, Rasotgi V, Jain S, Gupta V. Discovery of fifth serotype of dengue virus (DENV-5): A new public health dilemma in dengue control. Medical Journal Armed Forces India. 2015; 71(1): 67-70. doi: 10.1016/j.mjafi.2014.09.011

[4] Report of the meeting of the WHO/VMI workshop on dengue modeling. WHO/IVB/11.02. 2010. Available from: http://apps.who.int/iris/bitstream/10665/70625/1/WHO_IVB_11.02_eng.pdf

[5] Dengue vaccine: WHO position paper. WHO Weekly Epidemiological Record. 2016; 30(91): 349-364. Available from:www.who.int/wer

[6] Dengue guidelines for diagnosis, treatment, prevention and control. WHO. 2009. Available from: www.who.int/tdr/publications/documents/dengue-diagnosis.pdf?ua=1

[7] Chen YC, Cheng WF, Yang YC Yeh MK. Nanotechnologies Applied in Biomedical Vaccines. In: Stanciu SG, editor. Micro and Nanotechnologies for Biotechnology. INTECH, Croatia; 2016. p.85-105. doi: org/10.5772/63453

[8] Mahoney R, Chocarro L, Southern J, Francis DP, Vose J, Margolis H. Dengue vaccines regulatory pathways: A report on two meetings with regulators of developing countries. PLoS Medicine. 2011; 8(2): e1000418. doi: 10.1371/journal.pmed.1000418

[9] Guidelines for the clinical evaluation of dengue vaccines in endemic areas. WHO/IVB/08.12. 2008. Available from:apps.who.int/iris/bitstream/10665/69850/1/WHO_IVB_08.12_eng.pdf

[10] Ferguson NM, Rodríguez-Barraquer I, Dorigatti I, Mier-y-Teran-Romero L, Laydon DJ, Cummings DAT. Benefits and risks of the Sanofi-Pasteur dengue vaccine: Modeling Optimal Deployment. Science. 2016; 353(6303): 1033-1036. doi: 10.1126/science.aaf9590

[11] Aguiar M, Stollenwerk N, Halstead SB. The Impact of the newly licensed dengue vaccine in endemic countries. PLoS Neglected Tropical Diseases. 2016; 10(12): e0005179. doi: 10.1371/journal.pntd.0005179

[12] Scott LJ. Tetravalent Dengue Vaccine: A review in the prevention of dengue disease. Drugs. 2016; 76(13): 1301-1312. doi: 10.1007/s40265-016-0626-8.

[13] Abrão EP, Espósito DL, Lauretti F, da Fonseca BA. Dengue vaccines: what we know, what has been done, but what does the future hold? Revista De Saude Publica. 2015; 49: 60. doi: 10.1590/S0034-8910.2015049006146

[14] Thisyakorn U and Thisyakorn C. Latest developments and future directions in dengue vaccines. Therapeutic Advances in Vaccines. 2014; 2(1): 3-9. doi: 10.1177/2051013613507862

[15] Schmitz J, Roehrig J, Barrett A, Hombach J. Next generation dengue vaccines: a review of candidates in preclinical development. Vaccine. 2011; 29(42): 7276-7284. doi: 10.1016/j.vaccine.2011.07.017

[16] Edelman R, Durbin A, Roehrig JT, Smith PG, Hombach J, Farrar J. Long-term safety assessment of live attenuated tetravalent dengue vaccines: deliberations from a WHO technical consultation. Vaccine. 2013; 31(23): 2603-2609. doi: 10.1016/j.vaccine.2013.03.038

[17] López-Gatell H, Alpuche-Aranda CM, Santos-Preciado JI, Hernández-Ávila M. Dengue vaccine: local decisions, global consequences. 2016; 1; 94(11): 850-855. doi: 10.2471/BLT.15.168765

Chapter 8

Roadmap for the Introduction of a New Dengue Vaccine

Miguel Betancourt-Cravioto,
Jorge Abelardo Falcón-Lezama and
Roberto Tapia-Conyer

Additional information is available at the end of the chapter

http://dx.doi.org/10.5772/67745

"The impact of vaccination on the health of the world's people is hard to exaggerate. With the exception of safe water, no other modality has had such a major effect on mortality reduction and population growth"

Stanley Plotkin

Abstract

Dengue remains the most common vector-transmitted disease in the world despite enormous prevention and control efforts by endemic countries and regions. Today, after decades of research, public health programs contemplate as part of the intervention to control the disease, a safe and effective vaccine against dengue. In this chapter, we review general principles for developing a safe and efficacious vaccine against dengue virus, the current vaccine candidates approved and under research, and the roadmap for the introduction of a new dengue vaccine, based on the procedures, carried out by Mexico, for the licensure and eventual adoption of CYD-TDV vaccine, which concluded with Mexico becoming the first country in the world to grant licensure to a Dengue vaccine in December of 2015. Finally, we discuss the rationale for the adoption of dengue vaccines a public health policy and the paradigm shift required for the efficient adoption of vaccines in low- and middle-income countries.

Keywords: dengue control, vaccine, prevention, public health

1. Introduction

Vaccination is one of the most successful preventive measures in public health; its relevance for the prevention and control of infectious diseases is beyond any doubt. Vaccines have been paramount in the eradication of human and animal diseases such as smallpox [1] and rinderpest [2] and have been a main driver for the eradication efforts of other diseases (**Table 1**).

Disease	Main public health measures	Conclusion of the International Task Force for Disease Eradication
Dracunculiasis	Water sanitation, vector control, surveillance and contention	Eradicable
Lymphatic filariasis	Pharmacological treatment, vector control	Potentially eradicable
Measles	Vaccination	Potentially eradicable
Mumps	Vaccination	Potentially eradicable
Poliomyelitis	Vaccination	Eradicable
Rubella	Vaccination	Potentially eradicable
Taeniasis/cysticercosis	Improved sanitation, pharmacological treatment, vaccination of cattle	Potentially eradicable

Table 1. Candidate diseases for eradication. Modified from Ref. [3].

As we all know, in public health, disease eradication through vaccination is an ultimate goal; nonetheless, this is not the only benefit of vaccines. Well-documented advantages such as elimination of diseases, control of mortality, morbidity and complications of disease are positive impacts of immunizations. Additional benefits can be attributed to vaccines such as mitigation of disease severity, protection of unvaccinated population through herd immunity, prevention of antibiotic resistance, extension of life expectancy, enhancement of equality and empowerment of vulnerable populations. These effects are perhaps not as recognizable as disease eradication, but they have certainly shaped the health profile of entire populations [4].

Vector-transmitted diseases (VTDs) are a heterogeneous group of human illnesses caused by viral, bacterial and parasitic agents. Unlike many other infections in which transmission occurs directly between humans, VTD transmission cycles require the involvement of different arthropods such as mosquitoes, ticks, fleas, flies and kissing bugs, which work as vectors by carrying pathogens from humans to humans. In some VTDs like malaria, zika or dengue, arthropods and humans are the only components of the cycles; however, other VTDs like Chagas disease or Yellow fever are also zoonoses, which means that their transmission cycles include intermediate hosts, usually mammals. The more complex these cycles are, the more difficult VTDs control is [5], since more interventions are required to interrupt transmission. As an example, lymphatic filariasis is potentially eradicable since it has few vectors, and there is a non-expensive and effective treatment, which administered regularly to population at risk in large endemic areas ensures the interruption of transmission independently of vector circulation. Chagas disease, on the other hand, is considered non-eradicable since it has multiple vectors and hosts, it is difficult to diagnose, and the treatment is not well tolerated by most patients.

To date, prevention and control of VTDs, especially those transmitted by mosquitoes, rely mostly on vector control strategies, usually insecticide spraying and physical denial of vector's ecological niches. In the case of dengue, preventive measures include focal approaches with different schemes of insecticide use for indoor and outdoor settings aimed at larvae and adults, and the physical removal or destruction of mosquito breeding sites. For outbreak control, the same two interventions are usually applied with intensive schemes. For other VTDs, such as malaria, early identification and diagnosis of cases have proven to be an efficacious measure [6], but for a number of reasons such as cost, lack of point-of-care diagnostic tools and complicated logistics, this is not as applicable for dengue. Unfortunately, few vaccines have been developed successfully for this group of diseases, and nevertheless, examples such as the yellow fever vaccine show that, although challenging, vaccines can be essential for achieving or improving disease control. Thanks to the introduction of the vaccine, urban yellow fever is rare, and sylvatic yellow fever has been under control for decades.

Dengue virus (DENV) infection causes a broad spectrum of clinical manifestations ranging from asymptomatic infection to life-threatening severe dengue [7]. Each year, up to 390 million infections worldwide, resulting in about 96 million clinical cases, represent a huge burden of disease for health systems in endemic areas [8]. Although most cases are benign and only a minor fraction of these develop severe disease, the number of infections every year and consequently the number of severe forms of dengue continue to increase despite current vector control measures since there is no specific preventive measure focused on the host. The expenditure on vector control represents an enormous burden and a threat to health systems in low- and middle-income countries [9].

Climate change, urbanization and other anthropogenic factors facilitate transmission of dengue and other VTDs [10]. Current vector control strategies have not, with very few exceptions, provided the expected results in diminishing or stabilizing dengue transmission for long periods [11]. Case identification is not currently feasible and before the availability of dengue vaccines, no other preventive option existed for the host. Considering these perspectives, dengue vaccines are more than ever a true necessity for improving the health of the millions that inhabit dengue endemic regions.

2. Development of vaccines against dengue

Dengue virus (DENV) belongs to the *Flaviviridae* family. Vaccines against members of this family such as the yellow fever virus (YFV) [12], the Tick-borne Encephalitis virus (TBEV) [13], and the Japanese Encephalitis virus (JEV) [14] have been successfully developed; nonetheless, a reliable and efficacious vaccine against dengue remained an elusive goal for decades.

Some characteristics of the dengue virus and the disease it causes constitute a great challenge for the development of a dengue vaccine. Some of those related to the agent are the genotype divergence, which contrary to other members of the *Flaviviridae* family, is so wide that it translates into notable serotype divergence [15–17], therefore making difficult to identify immunogenic proteins that are widely conserved among serotypes. In the case of flaviviruses, the main immunogenic protein is located in the envelope (E protein), which as we will review below, it is the basis for the development of most of vaccine candidates against dengue.

Another important challenge lies in the pathophysiology of severe dengue, which is strongly associated with previous exposure to the dengue virus. A secondary exposure after initial "priming" is capable of triggering an exaggerated immune response characterized by a cytokine storm, which contributes to impaired endothelial function and plasma leakage as its main pathologic characteristic. Because of this, any vaccine developed against dengue needs to achieve a balance between being protective enough to prevent the disease and being sufficiently safe to avoid a pathologic immune response after priming [18].

An additional difficulty arises with the fact that a natural dengue infection elicits two types of antibodies. One type of antibodies is specific against the infecting serotype; these are usually long-lasting and with neutralizing capacity. The other type is cross-reactive to other serotypes, short lasting and non-neutralizing. Short lasting, non-neutralizing antibodies contribute to limit dengue epidemics and the number of serotypes that cause outbreaks. It is believed that in the long term, these non-neutralizing antibodies might play a role in the pathophysiology of dengue by facilitating the infection of larger number of cells during secondary exposures to the virus, a phenomenon called "antibody-dependent enhancement," or ADE [19]. Apparently, this phenomenon is not exclusive of dengue virus infections and has only been demonstrated in vitro; however, its real contribution to dengue pathophysiology is still under debate. Nonetheless, the risk of ADE needs to be taken into account when developing vaccines against dengue [20].

Based on these biological characteristics, it is desirable that any dengue vaccine developed be capable of immunizing simultaneously against each of its four known serotypes. Also, in order to avoid natural infections that might trigger secondary pathologic responses, the vaccine should be administered in a minimum-dose scheme and in a short period [21, 22]. Simulation studies have shown that even vaccines that do not elicit complete protection against all serotypes and require multiple-dose schemes would be valuable tools in the medium and long terms, since their positive impacts exceed the theoretical potential negative effects [23].

Table 2 shows a list of the most relevant vaccines against dengue, currently approved and under development. Although not a comprehensive list, we can observe the different types of vaccines, and as discussed below, their particular advantages and disadvantages. It is expected that in the near future, many of these vaccines will become available and will be introduced as part of national dengue control strategies in endemic countries and regions.

Vaccine	Manufacturer	Type	Serotypes included
CYD-TVD	Sanofi – Pasteur	Recombinant live-attenuated chimeric. PrM/E proteins cloned into a 17D YFV backbone	All four
DENVax	Takeda	Live attenuated. Recombinant PM/E proteins from DENV-1, DENV-3 and DENV-4 cloned into live-attenuated DENV-2	All four
TV003/TV005	NIAID/Butantan Institute	Live-attenuated admixture of mutated and chimeric viruses	All four
TDENV PIV	GSK	Purified, formalin-inactivated viruses	All four
V180	Merck	Recombinant subunit. Truncated E protein from each DENV serotype	All four
TVDV	NMRC	DNA. Plasmids encoding PrM/E genes	All four

Table 2. Vaccines currently used or under development against dengue [18, 22, 24, 25].

In general, live-attenuated vaccines are produced with viable viruses that have been modified from wild-type pathogenic viruses into less virulent or attenuated versions, which are unable to produce severe disease. They have the advantage of being capable of infecting cells and replicating, eliciting strong, long-term immune responses similar to natural infections. However, since these vaccines contain live viruses, reversion to pathogenic forms is always a possibility; therefore, surveillance is necessary to ensure the safety of the vaccine. These vaccines cannot be administered to pregnant women or immunosuppressed individuals [26]. The yellow fever and Japanese Encephalitis vaccines belong to this group.

Inactivated vaccines are produced by exposing a pathogenic agent to chemicals, heat, or radiation in a process called inactivation. These vaccines are preferred over live-attenuated vaccines due to the absence of risks such as reversion of virulence, or limitations on its usage in selected population groups such as pregnant women and immunosuppressed individuals. Although they are generally very stable, sometimes, the inactivation process alters the structure of the pathogens, and possibly the immunogenicity of the viral proteins, diminishing its efficacy to elicit a protective immune response. Given the alteration caused by the inactivation process, the viruses from these vaccines are unable to replicate, and therefore, the viral proteins must be highly immunogenic on their own. Otherwise, the vaccine formulation needs to be added with a booster or adjuvant to increase its immunogenicity. The formalin-inactivated TDENV-PIV dengue vaccine under development belongs to this group [26].

Subunit vaccines are similar to inactivated vaccines, but they are formulated with incomplete agents, usually proteins form the original pathogenic strain. Since they are not whole pathogens, they cannot replicate, and the risk of reversion is absent, but they also lack the immunogenicity of whole pathogens. Therefore, the trick is to reach an acceptable immunogenic capability with truncated proteins that are unable to be infectious [26]. The V180 dengue vaccine is being formulated using a subunit of the E protein.

Recombinant vector vaccines, also known as chimeric vaccines, are based on attenuated viruses or microbes to introduce DNA from a pathogenic agent mimicking a natural infection and stimulating the immune system. The CYD-TDV dengue vaccine is a live-attenuated chimeric tetravalent vaccine constructed by cloning DENV Pre-M and E genes into a yellow fever Virus 17D strain backbone and belongs to this group [27]. Phase 3 clinical trials have demonstrated the vaccine's efficacy in preventing severe forms of dengue and admissions to hospital [28–30]. WHO has published a position paper describing the recommended procedures and conditions under which this vaccine is to be used by the international community [31]. To date, this is the only existing approved vaccine in the world. It was first licensed in Mexico in December of 2015 [32], and by late 2016, 12 additional countries from Latin America and Southeast Asia have also granted licensure to CYD-TDV.

Finally, DNA vaccines are theoretically the safest type of vaccines. They are formed by nucleic acids that encode fragments of the original pathogenic agent that are administered directly into the cells in order to produce immunogenic proteins that provide a protective immune response against infection. Nonetheless, the immune response that these vaccines produce is usually weak, and although promising, they still are in experimental phases [26]. This strategy is used in the TVDV dengue vaccine, which relies on fragments of DENV prM/E proteins expressed by a plasmid vector.

3. The vaccine introduction process

Traditionally, the introduction of vaccines in low- and middle-income countries (LMIC) occurs years or even decades after they have been introduced in high-income countries. With very few exceptions, vaccines are usually developed, tested and adopted according to the public health needs of high-income countries. LMICs seldom participate in the vaccine development process and only uptake products already tested in developed markets.

Because of this passive behavior, it takes a long time for public health officials in LMICs to incorporate new vaccines since there is a tendency to wait for licensure, introduction and phase 4 studies in high-income countries before beginning the introduction process. This delay in the adoption of innovation in public health technologies causes unnecessary suffering for populations in need of such scientific advances to address their health needs.

Recent events such as the emergence of infectious diseases like zika and, chikungunya in the Americas, or the re-emergence of Ebola in Africa have exposed the weaknesses of public health systems, and the need to change this passive behavior in order to accelerate access to the benefits provided by vaccines for those who need them the most [33]. The aim is for LMICs to participate in all phases of vaccine development, from their theoretical conception to all levels of clinical trials, and then to reduce the elapsed time between the moment a safe and efficacious vaccine is ready for commercialization and the moment the vaccine is licensed and eventually adopted.

As an effort to promote the early adoption of vaccines in LMICs, the authors have pushed forward for a paradigm shift in the introduction of new vaccines by designing and supporting the implementation of a new strategy for vaccine introduction based on scientific and technical analyses, and the accompaniment of public health authorities in the process. The aim of this strategy is to modify the general attitude toward vaccine introduction by involving all relevant actors (government, academia, industry, National Regulatory Agencies, etc.) in a proactive and anticipatory exercise.

These efforts led to the development of a roadmap for the Introduction of New Vaccines that has been instrumented in Mexico for the incorporation of the new dengue vaccine. In the following section, we will describe the process followed to promote the early adoption of these novel vaccines as a public health policy in the country.

3.1. A roadmap for the introduction of a dengue vaccine

It is necessary to recognize that the process for the introduction of any vaccine does not begin with the development of a candidate molecule by researchers. This path actually starts with the daily activities of epidemiologists and public health workers in the field, which generate and provide reliable epidemiological information, thus revealing health needs characterized as disease cases, fatalities, stress to health systems or any other negative impact. In Mexico, as in many other countries, dengue has become a major challenge for public health in the last three decades causing large outbreaks, mortality, and an increase in the demand of health services across the country. Its seasonal and oscillatory behavior makes it difficult to predict when or where there will be outbreaks in order to anticipate control interventions.

http://dx.doi.org/10.5772/67745

As vaccine candidates developed by the pharmaceutical industry began to show results from early clinical trials in recent years suggesting the availability of a safe and efficacious dengue vaccine in the short term, the authors presented to Mexican Health authorities a roadmap proposal for the eventual adoption of such technologies into the Mexican context. This roadmap includes a series of well-defined steps to be followed in anticipation to the licensure of the vaccine by the National Regulatory Agency in order to be ready for early implementation.

To lead the anticipatory exercise, an independent, multidisciplinary body of experts, called Mexican Dengue Expert Group (MDEG), was specifically convened. The MDEG included representatives from academic and research institutions, public health authorities and representatives of the private and social sectors (**Figure 1**).

The objectives of the MDEG were to analyze and discuss all relevant aspects related to the possibility of the introduction in Mexico of the different vaccines under development and also to evaluate their potential impact on the disease epidemiology and the implications on the National Immunizations and Vector-Borne Disease Prevention and Control Programs, in order to issue recommendations to the Mexican Public Health Authorities.

The roadmap was presented to and accepted by national health authorities in Mexico, which accepted the MDEG as the group that would officially lead the process.

The specific topics discussed and analyzed by the MDEG were epidemiological data and burden of disease: economic and financial aspects, operational and logistical issues, legal and regulatory aspects, strategic communications and clinical issues (**Table 3**). All these elements were reviewed taking into account the available evidence on safety and efficacy of the different candidate vaccines.

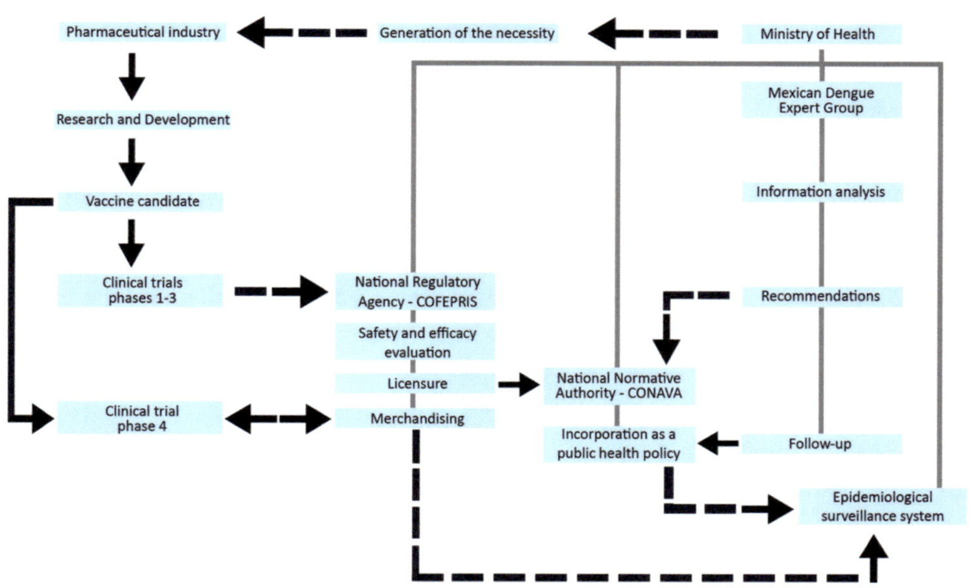

Figure 1. General roadmap for the introduction of a new dengue vaccine.

Subgroup of epidemiological information and disease burden

I. To define geographic areas for the introduction of a vaccine.
II. To define the target population.
III. To establish impact scenarios of the vaccination scheme.

Subgroup of economic and financial aspects

IV. To generate cost-benefit and cost-effective studies using modeling tools.
V. To define the budgetary requirements for the introduction of the vaccine into the country.

Subgroup of operational aspects

VI. To analyze the age groups for the application of the immunization scheme.
VII. To generate strategies and scenarios for vaccine application depending on the selected target population.
VIII. To discuss the relevance of strengthening the immunization information system in order to accurately measuring the coverage of the target population.
IX. To analyze the impact in the cold chain caused by the introduction of a new vaccine.
X. To develop the operational training strategy for the Universal Vaccination Program in the areas of vaccine introduction.

Subgroup of legal and regulatory aspects

XI. To ensure the readiness of the registration and licensure procedures for the vaccines.
XII. To orchestrate an automated pharmacosurveillance system to ensure the monitoring of adverse events following immunization (AEFI's) attributable to the vaccine introduction.

Subgroup of strategic communication

XIII. Generate strategies that allow the appropriate communication on the rationale behind a Dengue vaccine introduction to all relevant groups.
XIV. Develop specific communication channels for the new vaccine's target population.
XV. Ensure that messages on the general population inform on the importance of strengthening vector control, and the role of the new vaccine as part of an integral strategy, not as a substitute of prevention and control activities.

Subgroup of clinical aspects

XVI. Analyze the elements of clinical care in patients with Dengue that might result affected by the introduction of the vaccine.
XVII. Strengthen the health personnel capabilities in clinical scenarios for detecting and reporting AEFI.
XVIII. Strengthen the clinical personnel capacity for differential diagnosis of regional febrile diseases related to DF.

This figure describes the specific objectives from each working subgroup.

Table 3. Specific objectives for each subgroup in the Dengue Mexican Expert Group.

The roadmap included two phases. The first phase reviewed the existing evidence in order to analyze vaccine developments and the feasibility and requirements for the eventual adoption of such vaccines into the dengue control and immunization programs. This phase took place between 2011 and 2013 and resulted in an initial set of recommendations for the introduction of the vaccine in Mexico [34]. Evidence from a number of vaccine candidates in light of national epidemiological data quickly demonstrated that the adoption of any dengue vaccine in the future would require major improvements in many aspects.

With regard to epidemiological surveillance, the MDEG identified the need for strengthening the capacity of surveillance systems, networks, classification of cases and diagnostic protocols. Evidence of differential vaccine efficacy against the four dengue serotypes requires the improvement of virological typing and mathematical modeling capabilities to correctly evaluate the impact of vaccine introduction on the population.

Economic and financial issues were discussed as a basic element in the context of constrained resources such as those prevalent in LMICs; therefore, it was necessary to establish common methodologies for economic burden studies and those for cost-effectiveness of preventive and control interventions.

The analyses concerning the operational aspects required for the introduction of new vaccines concluded on the necessity for establishing baseline measurements to evaluate impact, feasibility of population selection from endemic areas with high risk of transmission and adoption of vaccines using currently available strategies in the country.

Regulatory issues were not essential before the beginning of the registration process; nonetheless, the MDEG was able to continuously review industry data, particularly results from phase II and III studies and also to participate in the development of post marketing surveillance systems that would be necessary in the event of the vaccine licensure.

Finally, social communication and health promotion had to be addressed in order to transmit clear messages on the safety and efficacy of vaccines, the implementation of vaccines into current integrated strategies for dengue control and not as an isolated intervention, and more important to clarify the regionalized strategy for these vaccines in contrast to universal vaccination schemes used regularly in the country.

After the first phase, the MDEG produced the following recommendations.

I. Strengthen epidemiologic, entomologic and virological surveillance and obtain data necessary for impact modeling of dengue vaccine introduction.

II. Carry out studies of the economic burden of dengue in Mexico, necessary for cost-benefit and cost-effectiveness analyses to support financial decisions.

III. Introduce the vaccine as soon as it becomes available.

IV. Invite potential vaccine producers to engage with the national regulatory authority to facilitate registration and licensing procedures.

V. Integrate the immunization schedule defined by the National Vaccination Council of Mexico and approved by COFEPRIS with pre-existing National Health Weeks.

VI. Define vaccination age groups according to epidemiologic risk and producers' recommendations.

VII. Collect data to support national information campaigns to facilitate introduction.

The second phase of the roadmap began in 2015 when the results from the phase 3 studies of the CYD-TDV vaccine were published and the licensure process for this vaccine by the Mexican National Regulatory Agency (COFEPRIS—National Commission for the Protection of Health Risks) began. The availability of these results raised the necessity for the MDEG to review the data derived from the CYD-TDV phase 3 trials [30], focusing on this occasion, on the analysis of the feasibility of introducing the vaccine as a public policy, considering the special characteristics of dengue as a disease and those of the vaccine as a preventive tool. As part of the work carried out in this phase, it was decided to incorporate an external perspective by extending an invitation to the Partnership for Dengue Control (PDC), an international organization integrated by world-class experts on dengue with the aim of supporting global elimination efforts for the disease, to participate in the proceedings. PDC experts participated actively in the discussions and issued specific recommendations that were included in the final document prepared by the MDEG.

After deep analysis of the available evidence, the MDEG presented to the Mexican Ministry of Health its final recommendations for the introduction of the dengue CYD-TDV vaccine [35]. The MDEG reiterated its support for the adoption of the vaccine and developed the criteria shown in **Table 4**.

In parallel, and recognizing the existence of a viable vaccine candidate, international institutions such as the World Health Organization began similar exercises, and in April of 2015, the Strategic Advisory Group of Experts on Immunization (SAGE) issued the first recommendations on the use of Dengue vaccines [36], which were followed by the emission of WHO's Position paper on dengue vaccination in July of 2016 [31]. These official documents recognize the availability of a licensed dengue vaccine and establish the conditions under which the introduction of CYD-TDV is to be considered. As observed, MDEG's recommendations are fully consistent with those issued by WHO, which consequently validate this innovative approach to vaccine introduction.

1. The following epidemiological criteria must be considered for the introduction of the new dengue vaccine into municipalities. At least four out of the six following conditions must be met:
    - **a.** Cumulative incidence above national mean during at least one of the last 5 years.
    - **b.** Notification of dengue confirmed cases for at least 20 continuous weeks in the immediate prior year.
    - **c.** Annual proportion of severe cases equal or above 1%, considering the total reported cases of severe dengue and dengue with warning signs.
    - **d.** At least one confirmed dengue fatality during the last 5 years.
    - **e.** Co-circulation of at least two serotypes, and/or circulation of serotype 3 and/or 4.
    - **f.** Seroprevalence above 60%.
2. To apply the vaccine on population aged 9, using current immunization strategies.
3. To use the three-dose immunization scheme established by the manufacturer.
4. To develop a communication strategy that allows informing the population on the adoption of this vaccine.
5. Logistic and operational aspects for the introduction of the vaccine must be guaranteed.
6. At the end of the first cohort, impact evaluation should be started.
7. Based on the previous points, the information generated by the MDEG, and its six subgroups will be sent to CONAVA for the feasibility analyses on the introduction of the dengue vaccine into the immunization scheme.

Table 4. MDEG recommendations for the introduction of a Dengue vaccine in Mexico.

The criteria developed by the MDEG cover epidemiological, operational and communication issues that are applicable to other endemic regions in the world. It is important to notice that additionally to seroprevalence, these criteria include other measurable health impacts such as cumulative incidence, outbreak duration, proportion of severe cases, fatalities and hyperendemicity. The inclusion of these effects grants flexibility to the decision-makers while considering or not the adoption of dengue vaccines taking into account the particular characteristics and resources of the region. Having additional criteria is an advantage, since seroprevalence studies are very expensive and time-consuming, while basic data on disease burden using confirmed cases are usually available for the vast majority of health systems.

Simultaneously to the anticipatory introduction exercise, the Mexican National Regulatory Agency (COFEPRIS—National Commission for the Protection of Health Risks) began the licensing process for the CYD-TDV dengue vaccine. As stated in international protocols, COFEPRIS followed a scrupulous evaluation process that included the vaccine's safety, efficacy and quality of the candidate vaccine and, according to the country's regulatory criteria. Although independent, these proceedings and those performed by the MDEG were not separately carried out, since representatives of the two bodies met regularly in order to feedback from each other's analyses. This feedback helped both parts to align their criteria, sources and information, and also contributed to optimize procedures while shortening the time for discussions. At the end of the registration processes, COFEPRIS issued a favorable resolution granting the licensure in December 2015 (**Figure 2**).

Having obtained the licensure for marketing the vaccine in the private sector, the next natural step is the procedure for the adoption of the vaccine as a health policy. It is now the responsibility of the National Vaccination Council (CONAVA—Consejo Nacional de Vacunación) to decide if, when and how to introduce the new dengue vaccine in Mexico. The final MDEG

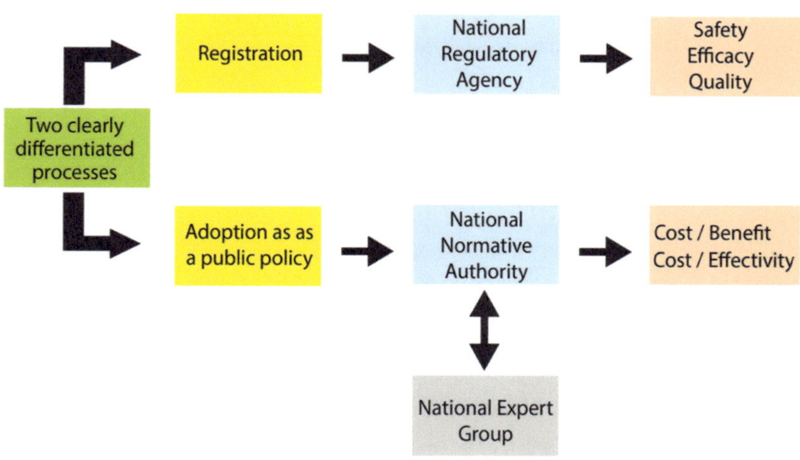
Registration
National Regulatory Agency
Safety Efficacy Quality
Two clearly differentiated processes
Adoption as as a public policy
National Normative Authority
Cost / Benefit Cost / Effectivity
National Expert Group

Figure 2. Processes of licensure and adoption as a public health policy.

recommendations were presented to the Council after the vaccine was licensed, and the proposed criteria were adopted as the basis for the document published as the interim policy regarding the CYD-TDV vaccine. The policy establishes a series of criteria for introduction of the vaccine by public health institutions (**Table 5**). At this point, the only remaining criterion to be fulfilled is the inclusion of CYD-TDV in the National Basic Catalogue of Medicinal Products, which has to be authorized by the General Health Council (Consejo de Salubridad General), the nation's top authority in Public Health matters.

The introduction of a tetravalent dengue vaccine as a public policy is to be considered under the following conditions:

I. To fulfill at least four, out of the following six epidemiological criteria:

   a. Population of states, municipalities or localities must have a demonstrable seroprevalence desirably equal or higher than 60%.

   b. Cumulative incidence above the national mean, during at least one of the last 5 years.

   c. Laboratory-confirmed cases of Dengue for at least 20 continuous weeks, during the last year.

   d. Annual proportion of severe dengue equal or higher than 1% considering total notified cases.

   e. At least one fatality recorded during the last 5 years.

   f. Co-circulation of at least two serotypes and/or circulation of serotype 3 and/or 4.

II. To be applied in population aged 9–16.

III. To be applied using a three-dose immunization scheme: 0, 6 and 12 months, subcutaneously.

IV. To ensure sufficient budget in order to guarantee the acquisition of the three-dose scheme for the cohorts to be immunized.

V. To guarantee financial capacity for logistics, human and operational resources for vaccine introduction.

VI. To develop a social communication strategy that allows informing the population on the introduction of this vaccine.

VII. To develop a nominal registry of vaccinated individuals, preferably with an electronic vaccination card.

VIII. The vaccine must be included in the Mexican basic catalogue of medicinal products.

IX. The vaccine will not be universally applied in the country.

X. States and social welfare institutions that wish to introduce the vaccine must define their strategies through their State Vaccination Councils, and present them to the national normative bodies for validation, in order to guarantee the compliance of the previously described conditions. Final approval must be obtained from the National Vaccination Council (CONAVA) and include all health institutions to comply with normative frame in order to guarantee notification and follow-up of adverse effects following immunization (AEFI), and the impact evaluation that includes cases, hospital admissions and averted deaths at the end of the first vaccination cohort. Vaccination strategy must be performed in a comprehensive manner, meaning that all public health institutions in the state should introduce the vaccine simultaneously.

XI. Seroprevalence studies for the target group are proposed, after assessing budgetary and operational feasibility.

XII. Resources for acquiring the vaccine must not be taken from the budget of the National Dengue Program or have any impact on the total budget allocated to health institutions, considering the budget of the year immediate prior to the vaccine introduction.

Table 5. National Vaccination Council's criteria for the introduction of a Dengue vaccine in Mexico [37].

http://dx.doi.org/10.5772/67745

4. Rationale for the adoption of a dengue vaccine as a public health policy

4.1. The paradigm shift

Existing epidemiological evidence shows that current surveillance and preventive and control measures are just not enough to reverse the currently increasing tendency of disease burden caused by DENV infection [8]. Newly recognized factors such as the contribution of human mobility on dengue transmission, its impact on control interventions [38] and the threats posed by the recent emergence of zika, chikungunya, and other VTDs are also important arguments to consider. To be able to curb the tendencies, vector control strategies need to evolve and adapt to new knowledge and technological developments in a way that has never occurred in the past but that is imperative in the face of the current challenges.

As discussed in this chapter, development and introduction of a dengue vaccine are a complex, challenging and demanding process for public health systems that requires the participation of all relevant actors. To finally have a safe and effective vaccine against this disease is a major breakthrough in the prevention and control of one of the most important VTD in the world, therefore, the necessity of health systems in endemic areas to be prepared for the adoption of this technology according to their particular needs and epidemiological characteristics.

Having achieved this milestone, the challenges now lie in operational aspects for the introduction into immunization schemes and public health strategies. Dengue vaccines have unique characteristics that make them different to other existing vaccines. For this reason it is required that health personnel and general public have access to complete reliable information to understand the indications, capacities and limitations of this vaccine, and more important, to recognize this tool as an integral piece of dengue control strategy. In order to facilitate this process, it is desirable to develop introduction guidelines for specific topics such as the vaccine, application procedures, surveillance, and mass communication among others.

As a theoretical argument, it is valid to expect that a vaccine is completely reliable, efficacious and safe, but in real life, vaccines are usually adopted considering a balance between positive and adverse effects. However, in reference to the development of this new vaccine, it has been recognized by leading experts in dengue that *"the era when most vaccines provided efficacy well beyond 90% is over. Many of the more recently developed vaccines only provide partial efficacy. Although vaccines are typically licensed on the basis of demonstrated efficacy, the ultimate goal of vaccination goes far beyond efficacy"* [39].

The availability of a licensed, safe and efficacious vaccine provides VTD prevention and control programs with a new tool to be added to the current arsenal. Vector control strategies should no longer be considered as the sole preventive measures for dengue control, and it must be acknowledged that the development of dengue vaccines constitutes an important milestone that needs to be thoroughly evaluated in scientific terms and not with dogmatic positions.

Unnecessary delays in the introduction of CYD-TDV or any other dengue vaccine will have important consequences for the population of endemic areas. The first and most obvious is the persistence of the current epidemiological trend with more and more people suffering from the disease and its consequences. Not introducing the vaccine will obstruct individuals from their right to obtain the protective benefits of the vaccine, benefits not currently provided by any other available measure.

Lacking hosts other than humans, being transmitted only by a specific and highly anthropophilic mosquito species, and being a predominantly urban disease, dengue elimination is theoretically feasible, but it requires a paradigm shift in prevention and control strategies that integrates additional approaches such as the introduction of a new vaccine to existing policies and approaches.

5. Conclusions

The use of vaccines has been critical in the control and eventual eradication of major epidemic diseases, especially those with direct transmission. Vaccines for VTDs such as the yellow fever vaccine have proven their value both as preventive tools and as control measures in the case of outbreaks.

The newly available dengue vaccine and those currently under development are valuable tools intended to complement, not replace, current and future dengue prevention and control strategies [40]. In the operational scope, this integration needs to be performed in a comprehensive manner in order to maximize the positive effects of individual measures [41], and to avoid the collateral effects of excessive usage of those currently available [42]. This approach will undoubtedly be essential for reaching the WHO's strategic goal of 25% reduction in morbidity and 50% reduction in mortality due to dengue by 2020 [43]. Delaying decisions regarding the introduction of dengue vaccines could have important public health and economic implications.

Just as with any other vaccine, the most important safety and efficacy evaluation will begin once it is used in a real-life environment, when the vaccine must demonstrate a measurable impact on the disease. This impact can be estimated through changes in age-stratified indicators such as total number of cases, incidence or lethality. Additionally, the introduction of a new vaccine needs to further evaluate its safety through pharmacosurveillance in order to identify any adverse effects attributable to the vaccine. With proper follow-up, it will be possible then to define the real usefulness of the vaccine as a public health measure.

As an exercise, the roadmap here described has provided valuable experiences and the expected results in a short period. The formation of National Expert Groups for the analysis of feasibility for the introduction of dengue vaccines was fundamental for achieving such goals and should be a requisite for any country willing to explore the adoption on any existing or future vaccines.

Acknowledgements

The authors wish to thank the representatives of the institutions that participated in The Mexican Dengue Expert Group (in strict alphabetical order):

Government institutions: Centro Nacional de Excelencia Tecnológica en Salud, Centro Nacional de Programas Preventivos y Control de Enfermedades, Centro Nacional para la Salud de la Infancia y la Adolescencia, Comisión Coordinadora de Instituto Nacionales de Salud y Hospitales de Alta Especialidad, Comisión Nacional para la Protección contra Riesgos Sanitarios, Dirección General de Calidad y Educación en Salud, Dirección General de Comunicación Social, Dirección General de Epidemiología, Instituto Nacional de Diagnóstico y Referencia Epidemiológicos, Dirección General de Promoción de la Salud, Hospital Infantil de México, Instituto de Seguridad Social y Servicios para los Trabajadores del Estado, Petróleos Mexicanos, Instituto Mexicano del Seguro Social, Instituto Nacional de Ciencias Médicas y Nutrición "Salvador Zubirán," Instituto Nacional de Pediatría, Instituto Nacional de Salud Pública, Servicios de Salud de la Ciudad de México, Servicios de Salud de Nuevo León, Servicios de Salud de Tamaulipas, Servicios de Salud de Veracruz, Unidad de Análisis Económico—Secretaría de Salud.

Academic and research institutions: Centro de Investigación y Estudios Avanzados, Instituto Politécnico Nacional, Universidad Autónoma Metropolitana, Universidad Nacional Autónoma de México.

Social and private sectors: Fundación Carlos Slim, Sociedad Mexicana de Salud Pública A. C.

Author details

Miguel Betancourt-Cravioto*, Jorge Abelardo Falcón-Lezama and Roberto Tapia-Conyer

*Address all correspondence to: mbetancourt@fundacioncarlosslim.org

Carlos Slim Foundation, México City, Mexico

References

[1] World Health Organization. Resolution of the Thirty-third World Health Assembly. Available in: http://www.zero-pox.info/who_other/WHA33-R3.pdf [Accessed: 2016-12-16].

[2] World Organisation for Animal Health. Declaration of global eradication of rinderpest and implementation of follow-up measures to maintain world freedom from rinderpest. Available in: http://www.oie.int/fileadmin/Home/eng/Media_Center/docs/pdf/RESO_18_EN.pdf [Accessed: 2016-12-16].

[3] The Carter Center. Diseases considered for global eradication by the international task force for disease eradication. Available in: https://www.cartercenter.org/resources/pdfs/news/health_publications/itfde/updated_disease_candidate_table.pdf [Accessed: 2016-12-16].

[4] Andre FE, Booy R, Bock HL, Clemens J, Datta SK, John TJ, et al. Vaccination greatly reduces disease, disability, death and inequity worldwide. Bull World Health Org. 2008;86:140-6.

[5] World Health Organization. A global brief on vector-borne diseases. 2014. Available in: http://apps.who.int/iris/bitstream/10665/111008/1/WHO_DCO_WHD_2014.1_eng.pdf [Accessed: 2016-12-16].

[6] Gosling J, Case P, Tulloch J, Chandramohan D, Wegbreit J, Newby G, et al. Effective program management: a cornerstone of malaria elimination. Am J Trop Med Hyg. 2015;93(1):135-8. doi:10.4269/ajtmh.14-0255

[7] World Health Organization. Dengue Guidelines for diagnosis, treatment, prevention and control, Geneve. 2009. Available in: http://www.who.int/tdr/publications/documents/dengue-diagnosis.pdf?ua=1 [Accessed: 2016-12-16].

[8] Bhatt S, Gething PW, Brady OJ, Messina JP, Farlow AW, Moyes CL, et al. The global distribution and burden of dengue. Nature. 2013;496(7446):504-7. doi:10.1038/nature12060 PMID: 23563266

[9] Shepard DS, Undurraga EA, Halasa YA, Stanaway JD. The global economic burden of dengue: a systematic analysis. Lancet Infect Dis. 2016;16(8):935-41. doi:10.1016/S1473-3099(16)00146-8

[10] Rochlin I, Faraji A, Ninivaggi DV, Barker CM, Kilpatrick AM. Anthropogenic impacts on mosquito populations in North America over the past century. Nat Commun. 2016;7:13604. doi:10.1038/ncomms13604

[11] Achee NL, Gould F, Perkins TA, Reiner RC Jr, Morrison AC, Ritchie SA, et al. A critical assessment of vector control for dengue prevention. PLoS Negl Trop Dis. 2015;9(5):e0003655. doi:10.1371/journal.pntd.0003655

[12] Theiler M, Smith HH. The use of yellow fever virus modified by in vitro cultivation for human immunization. J Exp Med. 1937;31;65(6):787-800.

[13] Kunz C, Hofmann H, Stary A. Field studies with a new tick-borne encephalitis (TBE) vaccine. Zentralbl Bakteriol Orig A. 1976;234(1):141-4.

[14] Okuno Y, Okamoto Y, Yamada A, Baba K, Yabuuchi H. Effect of current Japanese encephalitis vaccine on different strains of Japanese encephalitis virus. Vaccine. 1987;5(2):128-32.

[15] Heinz FX, Stiasny K. Flaviviruses and flavivirus vaccines. Vaccine. 2012;30:4301-6. doi:10.1016/j.vaccine.2011.09.114

[16] Wahala WM, Donaldson EF, de Alwis R, Accavitti-Loper MA, Baric RS, de Silva AM. Natural strain variation and antibody neutralization of dengue serotype 3 viruses. PLoS Pathog. 2010;6:e1000821. doi:10.1371/journal.ppat.1000821

[17] Ecker M, Allison SL, Meixner T, Heinz FX. Sequence analysis and genetic classification of tick-borne encephalitis viruses from Europe and Asia. J Gen Virol. 1999;80(Pt 1): 179-85.

[18] Vannice KS, Roehrig JT, Hombach J. Next generation dengue vaccines: A review of the preclinical development pipeline. Vaccine. 2015;33(50):7091-9. doi:10.1016/j.vaccine.2015.09.053

[19] Endy TP, Nisalak A, Chunsuttitwat S, Vaughn DW, Green S, Ennis FA, et al. Relationship of preexisting dengue virus (DV) neutralizing antibody levels to viremia and severity of disease in a prospective cohort study of DV infection in Thailand. J Infect Dis. 2004;189(6):990-1000. doi:10.1086/382280

[20] Moi ML, Takasaki T, Kurane I. Human antibody response to dengue virus: implications for dengue vaccine design. Trop Med Health. 2016;44:1. doi:10.1186/s41182-016-0004-y

[21] Flipse J, Smit JM. The complexity of a dengue vaccine: a review of the human antibody response. PLoS Negl Trop Dis. 2015;9(6):e0003749. doi:10.1371/journal.pntd.0003749

[22] Lim SK, Lee YS, Namkung S, Lim JK, Yoon IK. Prospects for dengue vaccines for travelers. Clin Exp Vaccine Res. 2016;5(2):89-100. doi:10.7774/cevr.2016.5.2.89

[23] Rodriguez-Barraquer I, Mier-y-Teran-Romero L, Schwartz IB, Burke DS, Cummings DA. Potential opportunities and perils of imperfect dengue vaccines. Vaccine. 2014;32(4):514-20. doi:10.1016/j.vaccine.2013.11.020

[24] Schwartz LM, Halloran ME, Durbin AP, Longini IM Jr. The dengue vaccine pipeline: Implications for the future of dengue control. Vaccine. 2015;33(29):3293-8. doi:10.1016/j.vaccine.2015.05.010

[25] Liu Y, Liu J, Cheng G. Vaccines and immunization strategies for dengue prevention. Emerg Microbes Infect. 2016;5(7):e77. doi:10.1038/emi.2016.74

[26] Clem AS. Fundamentals of Vaccine Immunology. J Global Infect Dis. 2011;3(1):73-8. doi:10.4103/0974-777X.77299

[27] Guy B, Barrere B, Malinowski C, Saville M, Teyssou R, Lang J. From research to phase III: preclinical, industrial and clinical development of the Sanofi Pasteur tetravalent dengue vaccine. Vaccine. 2011;29(42):7229-41. doi:10.1016/j.vaccine.2011.06.094

[28] Capeding MR, Tran NH, Hadinegoro SR, Ismail HI, Chotpitayasunondh T, Chua MN, et al. Clinical efficacy and safety of a novel tetravalent dengue vaccine in healthy children in Asia: a phase 3, randomised, observer-masked, placebo-controlled trial. Lancet. 2014;384(9951):1358-65. doi:10.1016/S0140-6736(14)61060-6

[29] Villar L, Dayan GH, Arredondo-Garcia JL, Rivera DM, Cunha R, Deseda C, et al. Efficacy of a tetravalent dengue vaccine in children in Latin America. N Engl J Med. 2015;372(2):113-23. doi:10.1056/NEJMoa1411037

[30] Hadinegoro SR, Arredondo-Garcia JL, Capeding MR, Deseda C, Chotpitaya-sunondh T, Dietze R, et al. Efficacy and long-term safety of a dengue vaccine in regions of endemic disease. N Engl J Med 2015;373(13):1195-206. doi:10.1056/NEJMoa1506223

[31] World Health Organization. Dengue vaccine: WHO position paper – July 2016. Weekly Epidemiological record. 2016;30(91):349-64. Available in: http://www.who.int/wer/2016/wer9130.pdf?ua=1 [Accessed: 2016-12-16].

[32] Comisión Federal para la Protección contra Riesgos Sanitarios. Press Release, December 9, 2015. Available in: http://www.cofepris.gob.mx/Documents/NotasPrincipales/09122015.pdf [Accessed: 2015-12-16].

[33] World Health Organization. Final trial results confirm Ebola vaccine provides high protection against disease. Press release December 23, 2016. Available in: http://www.who.int/mediacentre/news/releases/2016/ebola-vaccine-results/en/ [Accessed: 2017-01-06].

[34] Betancourt-Cravioto M, Kuri-Morales P, González-Roldán JF, Tapia-Conyer R; Mexican Dengue Expert Group. Introducing a dengue vaccine to Mexico: development of a system for evidence-based public policy recommendations. PLoS Negl Trop Dis. 2014;8(7):e3009. doi:10.1371/journal.pntd.0003009

[35] Betancourt-Cravioto M, Falcón-Lezama JA, Kuri-Morales P, Gonzalez-Roldan JF, Tapia-Conyer R, and the Mexican Dengue Expert Group. Introducing a dengue vaccine to Mexico part II: A roadmap for the introduction and final recommendations (manuscript in preparation, 2017).

[36] World Health Organization. Summary of the April 2016 meeting of the Strategic Advisory Group of Experts on Immunization (SAGE). Available in: http://www.who.int/immunization/sage/meetings/2016/april/SAGE_April_2016_Meeting_Web_summary.pdf?ua=1 [Accessed: 2017-01-06].

[37] Sociedad Mexicana de Salud Pública A. C. Press Release on CONAVA recommendations concerning the introduction of a new dengue vaccine. Available in: http://smsp.org.mx/docs/vacuna_dengue.pdf [Accessed: 2016-12-16].

[38] Falcón-Lezama JA, Martínez-Vega RA, Kuri-Morales PA, Ramos-Castañeda J, Adams B. Day-to-day population movement and the management of dengue epidemics. Bull Math Biol. 2016;78(10):2011-33. doi:10.1007/s11538-016-0209-6

[39] Wilder-Smith A, Vannice KS, Hombach J, Farrar J, Nolan T. Population perspectives and World Health Organization recommendations for CYD-TDV dengue vaccine. J Infect Dis. 2016;214(12):1796-9. doi:10.1093/infdis/jiw341

[40] World Health Organization. Handbook for integrated vector management. Geneva, Switzerland: World Health Organization; 2012. Available in: http://www.who.int/iris/handle/10665/44768 [Accessed: 2016-12-16].

[41] PAHO/WHO/AMEXCID, Editors. Mesoamerican Master Plan for the Integrated Management of Dengue and Chikungunya Prevention and Control May, 2015. Available in: http://www.proyectomesoamerica.org/joomla/images/Documentos/Proyectos/Salud/Master%20Plan%20Dengue.pdf [Accessed: 2016-12-16].

[42] Centers for Disease Control and Prevention. Information on aerial spraying. Available in: https://www.cdc.gov/zika/vector/aerial-spraying.html [Accessed: 2016-12-16].

[43] World Health Organization. Global Strategy for dengue prevention and control. Geneve, 2012-2020. Available in: http://apps.who.int/iris/bitstream/10665/75303/1/9789241504034_eng.pdf [Accessed: 2016-12-16].